A LETTER TO THE READER

"Not to volunteer aid when unintentional suicide is going on seems nothing less than criminal."
                    DR. EDWARD HOOKER DEWEY

Dear Friend of Healthful Living,

Would you believe me if I told you that UNINTENTIONAL SUICIDE *IS* GOING ON IN AMERICA? That, *IN FACT*, 98½% of ALL Americans suffer from some debilitating physical derangement, impairment or disease? And, though we spend over 90 billion dollars annually *ON DISEASE*, ALMOST NOTHING is being spent or done CONSTRUCTIVELY to bring Americans to a state of fine health?

And would you believe me if I stated that vigorous robust health, *completely disease free, IS* the *NORMAL* STATE of human existence through a rewarding life *greatly in excess of 100 years?*

Would you believe me if I assured you that, with the knowledge we have today and especially as found in the astonishingly SIMPLE but *TRUE* health system of NATURAL HYGIENE, *NO ONE* need suffer any form of disease, illness, ailment, or malady? (Absolutely nothing! No colds, no headaches, no indigestion, no dental cavities, no constipation OR ANYTHING ELSE! A thoroughly hygienic life makes this possible.)

Would you believe me if I say that *we can* create a condition of general health in America that would relegate almost all ACHES, PAINS, AILMENTS AND DISEASES TO THE ASHCAN OF HUMAN HISTORY?

I know this sounds so incredible that you do not believe me. This is understandable. Under the pernicious notions fostered about health by the mis-educated and by profit-motivated interests which dominate our society we simply cannot persuade ourselves that exuberant good health, COMPLETELY DISEASE-FREE, is possible for all OR EVEN FOR OURSELVES!

I invite you—I URGE YOU—to conscientiously investigate the NATURAL HYGIENE program for wonderful health—FOR YOUR SAKE—*FOR AMERICA'S SAKE!*

Yours for health and happiness,
T. C. FRY
for NATURAL HYGIENE

PROGRAM FOR
DYNAMIC HEALTH

AN INTRODUCTION TO NATURAL HYGIENE

•

*The only
true health system*

•

T. C. FRY

NATURAL HYGIENE PRESS
A Division of
AMERICAN NATURAL HYGIENE SOCIETY, INC.
1920 Irving Park Road
Chicago, Illinois 60613
A Not for Profit Educational Organization

- NATURAL HYGIENE is a simple health system that is in harmony with nature, in accord with the principles of vital organic existence, correct in science, sound in philosophy, in agreement with common sense and successful in practice.

- NATURAL HYGIENE employs strictly natural means for attaining and maintaining ideal health.

- NATURAL HYGIENE is a health care system that makes possible a long happy rewarding life, *completely free* of diseases.

- NATURAL HYGIENE is a way of life and has nothing in common with the so-called healing arts. NATURAL HYGIENE holds that the organism is self-sufficient if supplied with its requirements, that is, fresh air, pure water, sunshine, exercise, wholesome foods, rest, sleep, security of life and its means, etc. NATURAL HYGIENE rejects all drugs, medications and treatments, holding that they interfere with vital processes and are most often downright injurious. NATURAL HYGIENE recognizes the plainly obvious in asserting that only the living organism can heal itself if injured or diseased. The AMERICAN NATURAL HYGIENE SOCIETY is, therefore, devoted to teaching people how to live correctly, i.e., in accord with their biological heritage.

Printing History
First Printing, June 1974
ISBN-0-914532-08-1
Copyright N.H.P. 1974
Library of Congress Number: 74-82366

TABLE OF CONTENTS

	page
Dedication	1
In Tribute	1
A Hope and an Invitation	2
On Understanding	2
How the Author Discovered NATURAL HYGIENE	3
Some Illuminating Thoughts on Truth and Health	12
Why This Volume Had to Be Written	16
Are Americans Really a Healthy People?	17
America's Desperate Need for a Valid Health System	22
The Essence of NATURAL HYGIENE	27
An Elaboration upon Eighteen Factors and Influences Essential to Superb Health and Wellbeing	33
What Is NATURAL HYGIENE?	48
Fasting as a Part of Your Health Program	52
How You Can Enjoy Superb Health—Your Daily Program for Wellbeing	63
Obtaining Nutritious Food	69
The Proper Foods to Eat	70
Combining Foods Properly	72
Food Combining Guide	74

Diet Principles to Follow That Do Not Cause Acid Indigestion, Upset Stomach, Constipation, Heartburn, Digestive Disorders	75
How to Increase the Nutritional Value of Your Food Several Hundred Per Cent by a Simple Change in the Way You Eat It	80
Why You Should Not Eat Bread—Any Kind	82
Why Babies Should Not Be Fed Cereals	83
Why Salt Should Never Be Used	85
How to Increase Your Brainpower and Mental Alertness	90
A Simple Test You Can Make to Determine Your State of Health	92
Questions and Answers on NATURAL HYGIENE	95
How Over 200 Million Americans Are Hooked on Drugs and Don't Realize It	98
Do Drugs or "Medicines" Really Cure?	107
Cures! Cures! Cures!	109
Is NATURAL HYGIENE Scientific?	116
How, by Following the NATURAL HYGIENE Program, the Average Family Can Save Over $2,000 Yearly	117

DEDICATION

I dedicate this book to the world's misled millions who seek happiness and well-being but who know not how to find it. I humbly consecrate the collected knowledge of this volume to a suffering people in the hope they will welcome and embrace its essential message, thus freeing themselves of the shackles of disease foisted upon them by the errant, the profit-motivated commercial interests that do not care about the consequences to health of those who use their pernicious products and the gain-motivated traffickers in human disease.

IN TRIBUTE

I owe a profound debt of gratitude to DR. HERBERT M. SHELTON of San Antonio, Texas, the greatest genius the health movement has ever known. Without the inspiration and guidance of his vast knowledge and understanding I would be unable to bring this information to you as I would still share the misconceptions, the ignorance, the despair and the suffering almost all Americans endure.

If America survives the debauchery of its death dealing "food", medical and drug trusts, it will owe its survival largely to Dr. Shelton!

A HOPE AND AN INVITATION

I hope this little volume will be instrumental in introducing to you and to America, indeed, the peoples of the world, a true health philosophy and practice that will enable them to realize the high potential which millions of years of development endowed them.

You're invited to help the American Natural Hygiene Society in distributing this inexpensive volume far and wide.

ON UNDERSTANDING

It has been observed that an ounce of prevention is worth a pound of cure. It could just as truly be said that it's worth a ton of cure for, in health, nature forgives no transgressions of her immutable principles. Every act contrary to the principles of health has its bad physiological consequences and cannot be undone. Every practice in accord with the fundamental principles of health as outlined herein has its beneficial results.

I submit that an ounce of understanding is better than a pound of knowledge and that a pound of knowledge is worth a ton of belief. I bid you, therefore, seek understanding above all things.

How the Author Discovered Natural Hygiene, His Experience and How He Practices It

Your writer has been on the Natural Hygiene regimen for just over three years.

In late 1970 when I made *my* GREAT HEALTH DISCOVERY in the form of DR. HERBERT M. SHELTON'S fine book, SUPERIOR NUTRITION, I was very conformistic in my living practices.

At that time eating was not, for me, for the sole function of nourishing the body. Gourmandizing was one of my hobbies! In pursuit of the pleasures of what I now realize was a perverted and depraved taste I ate indiscriminately as long as eating was a "taste delight" and I never stopped to think about the purpose of eating or the consequences that might result.

I discovered Dr. Shelton's fine book on a holiday in 1970 among some of the many books I had purchased nearly 16 years earlier. I now regard much of my life as being LOST, especially the nearly 16 years in which I possessed the open sesame to superb health! I read SUPERIOR NUTRITION completely on the day of its discovery. I reread it within a week, marking it liberally where I found its contents to be nothing less than revelations for me.

So inspiring and so very obviously true was this book, that from that day to this I have not:

- Partaken of meat, fish, eggs, milk or any other animal food.
- Used a particle of salt, pepper, spices, mustard, sauces, catsup or any other condiment.
- Eaten or partaken of breads, chocolates, candies, ice creams, pastries or any of hundreds of other concoctions that are popular.
- Drank of teas, coffees, alcoholics or any other beverage than pure distilled water!
- Taken any drugs, shots, pain killers, sleeping pills, aspirins, antacid pills or concoctions, "medicines", or any other injurious substances.
- Eaten but very little cooked foods!

Subsequently I stopped using soaps (cleansing is a mechanical, not a chemical process!), toothpastes, deodorants, shampoos, shaving creams, skin cleansers, lotions and other cosmetics!

I undertook most of these radical changes in my life IN A SINGLE DAY! So heavily did the truths of Dr. Shelton's book weigh upon me! I had always regarded myself as a creature of truth and it was beholden upon me to follow its dictates *upon discovery!*

So astounded was my family by this revolutionary turnabout in my regimen they thought I had gone kooky!

At 5 feet 6½ inches in height I was a hefty 195 to 198 pounds. I had a whole catalog of ailments and frequent bouts with colds and "viruses". At 44 years of age I had pimples, blackheads, twitching of the eyes, heavy dandruff, perpetual indigestion, migraine headaches, acid stomach, frequent colds, "malarial attacks", dental cavities, defective vision (I wore glasses but no longer do!), continual sluggishness and tiredness, constipation, sinus troubles, angina pectoris (heart pains), bad breath, foul stools, obnoxious body odors, a runny nose, continual mucus expectoration, rheumatic or arthritic joints and other complaints. I had a "normal" pulse of 70 to 75 versus a normal pulse today of 44 to 48!

Going on a completely living food diet consisting exclusively of certain vegetables, fruits, nuts and seeds caused the most startling changes to occur. There was a disappearance of one complaint after another! My weight dropped so rapidly it was frightening. I lost twenty pounds within the first three weeks. Then I undertook a five day fast during which I suffered the tortures of the damned (a 5-day fast occasions no discomfort whatsoever now—nothing more than a mild hunger on the first day). During my first fast every complaint I ever had seemed to revisit me all at once though, in reality, such was not the case. On this five day fast I lost another ten pounds. My wife became concerned. My size 44 coats, size 40 waisted pants and size 17 necked shirts were so unfilled that I was characterized as a walking skeleton! My face which had been so full, *bloated* in fact, was becoming thin, haggard and sallow in appearance.

Despite the importunities of wife, relatives and friends I not only stuck with the diet but started an exercise program!

The first day I started to run around my block (630 yards) I couldn't manage more than 400 before I was on the verge of collapse. It took me a week of practice to make it around on one try. Today I can run around the block six to eight times and still go through a heavy regimen of other activities and then go to work —in fact THIS IS my daily practice now.

After about three months on the new living food diet (nothing cooked or processed in any way! I ate fresh foods in the *NATURAL STATE* just as nature delivered them from the garden or farm) and with intermittent fasts I was down to 144 pounds. Dr. Shelton had stated that drastic weight loss would be the case. Expecting this I was rather pleased though sometimes worried.

I remained at 144 pounds a few days and then something happened to me—a kind of euphoria! A new sparkle was in my eyes, noticeably so. My skin color changed. My eyes which had looked a glassy yellow and somewhat bloodshot now became white.

My wife who was on the verge of summoning a doctor against my wishes noticed the sharp change. Within a week my weight was back up to 148 on the very same diet and a month later I was around 155 pounds where it has remained almost continously ever since.

All my complaints have disappeared! My hair is still mostly gray but my balding has definitely stopped. I haven't had a single cold! No "malarial attacks" have put in an appearance. My nose no longer runs! My headaches have never recurred since my third fast (a fast brought on headaches and nausea at first). I would say that, at 47, my health is as fine as it could be after the damage I suffered through 44 years of wrong living!

A typical day begins for me at 5:00 A.M. to 6:00 A.M. I arise and begin my first daily ablution. This is a scalp massage with a rubber fingered instrument. I give my head a dry cleaning as I do not wash my hair except on rare occasions. Though somewhat gray there is a luster to my hair and it always appears clean and "fresh washed". This first step in my day's activities brings me to a high state of awareness. Then I don athletic shorts or a sweat suit. My first activity is on a chinning bar. I do 12 to 15 continuous chin ups. This really *awakens* me! When I started my regimen I could barely manage four chinups. Then I set off jogging. This gradually increases until I have traversed 400 to 500 yards whereupon I find myself running rather than jogging. I usually run around the block for three times, just over a mile, unless I have a pair of ankle weights on in which case I rarely run more than twice around.

Upon return to my abode I go through an array of exercises—body twists, head and eye exercises, jumping jacks, pushups, body bends, knee bends, weight lifting, pull ups, etc. I spend perhaps 35 to 40 minutes going through my exercise program. During this time I always build up perspiration, even on the coldest winter day, and I get lots of deep breathing as required by my intense activity.

After my exercise program I enter a warm shower where I gradually increase the water temperature until it is perhaps a few degrees warmer than body temperature—never uncomfortable. I use a flesh brush only. I never use soap. Cleansing is a mechanical, not a chemical process. Toward the end of the shower, I gradually make the water cool but never unpleasantly so.

After my shower I rinse my mouth and teeth with water. I do not use either a toothbrush or toothpaste. A mouthful of chemicals are actually harmful. I haven't had any new cavity since going on my program! Moreover, I do not have bad breath. Bad breath is born of an unclean internal system and rarely originates in the mouth except in the case of rotting teeth, gums or material allowed to remain and decompose in the mouth.

My daily shave then takes place and I perform this act with only a brush and a razor. The shower has wettened my face and it is only necessary to wetten it slightly more with the brush. I get just as comfortable and just as close a shave as I ever did.

After shaving I usually lie down for about 15 to 20 minutes. This little relaxation seems to be the topping that makes for a great day.

After arising from this little rest I either read or undertake some chores, perhaps gardening. Around 8:00 AM I depart for the office where I usually work until 5:00 PM. Of the five days I am at the office I usually eat a noon meal not more than three times. Actually, I am fasting every Monday and automatically miss this noon meal every week. My first meal of the day is usually a light fruit meal, usually of a single kind, rarely more than two kinds. My first meal is of a fruit with high water content such as grapes, melon, peaches, pears, apples, bananas, etc. With grapes I may have some raisins. In the summer I usually eat only a high water content fruit meal whereas in the winter I may have bananas only or some dates, raisins or figs along with some high water content fruit. My water requirements are very low in the winter and I find it necessary to drink water ONLY on those days when I fast.

I return home after the day's work and relax about half an hour with my newspaper or the day's mail. My evening meal is usually partaken around 6:30 to 7:00 and lasts for about an hour! I eat rather slowly and I masticate my food thoroughly. Most of my eating time is occupied by two or three vegetables, usually greens, which I eat heavily. NONE OF MY FOOD IS COOKED! I try to eat in as airy a place as possible, even outdoors except when the temperature is too low to permit. My vegetables are thoroughly washed and are organically grown where possible. On occasion at least one of them are either alfalfa or mung bean sprouts.

The "main course" of my evening meal can be a number of rather concentrated foods but I find myself more often eating three or four ounces of sunflower seeds, three or four ounces of nuts, usually almonds, pecans, filberts (hazel nuts), brazil nuts or coconut. I sometimes eat sesame seeds (whole!), squash seeds and, on rare occasions, peanuts. About a third of my evening meals are starch meals and my favorite starch meal is one or two sweet potatoes uncooked and unpeeled.

After my evening meal I again relax for about half an hour in my music room. Then I take up reading, music appreciation, writing, responding to mail or do some office work I have brought home. Most of my evenings are spent in part with my family. Once a week I play chess. I play chess after a day of fasting on Monday evenings as I can play better by far after having missed a day of meals.

I usually retire about 11:00 PM though I retire earlier or later on occasions, whenever sleepiness overtakes me. I sleep in a *very soft* bed in a room made as airy or as well ventilated as possible. Constant fresh air helps the body to assimilate, regenerate and eliminate faster, hence makes the sleep sounder and reduces the time needed for sleep.

I follow a 10 to 12 meal a week plan. From Sunday evening until Tuesday noon I fast and, about every month or so extend the fast to three or more days. I never eat my first meal (breakfast, that is, the meal that *breaks* the *fast*) until about noon which can be as early as 11:00 AM or as late as 1:30 PM. I usually skip the noon meal if not eaten by 1:30 PM. Business circumstances or a lack of hunger may deny me the noon meal. If I eat a full week of meals they number not more than 12.

As I write this I suffer no complaints except lingering gray hair which I've had for nearly ten years. Being thoroughly cognizant of the fine results of my regimen through better and greater performance, a wonderful feeling and better disposition, a happy lack of ailments and "viruses", I find it no drag or in any way a problem to follow the hygienic program I've established.

I can recommend nothing better than the establishment and diligent pursuit of the hygienic program of living!

Some Illuminating Thoughts on Truth and Health

"Truth is my handmaiden, Wherever she leads, there will I go."

"Nothing is so easy as to deceive one's self; for what we wish, that we readily believe." DEMOSTHENES

"Our most unforgiveable sin is to reject and denounce that which we do not readily understand or which is contrary to our acquired habits and outlook."

"Better to be ignorant than to have learned so much that isn't so."

"In light of the incredible ease and simplicity of always being healthy, the person who becomes sick should be ashamed of himself."

"The greatest danger in all disease lies in the treatment of it, not in the sickness itself." after PURINTON

"Good health ends three fourths of life's miseries." MITCHELL

"It has always been one of the most difficult practical problems in the world to present new truths so as not to offend old errors; for persons are very apt to regard arguments directed against their opinions as attacks upon their persons; and many there are who mistake ingrained prejudices for established principles." DR. RUSSELL THACKER TRALL

"The most formidable weapon against errors of every kind is reason." THOMAS PAINE

"A suffering body cripples its mind also." J.H. TILDEN M.D.

"Convince a man against his will, he remains of the same opinion still." SCHOPENHAUER

"Make yesterday's finalities today's question marks. Make today's finalities tomorrow's question marks."

"But I ask no reader to take anything in this book as truth merely because I have put it into the book. I ask, instead, that my readers think, investigate, test and find out for themselves whether what I say is true or false. Take no man as your guide. Truth alone should guide you. If I speak not truth, if I err, if I am wrong, cast aside what I say and seek elsewhere. *Mistake not authority for truth, but make truth your authority.*" DR. HERBERT SHELTON in SUPERIOR NUTRITION.

"The use of the word "believe" is a confession of ignorance. We do not employ the word where we have knowledge and it is not necessary to believe that which we know."

"The body is self-correcting. Give the body a prolonged rest (fast) and it will perform a general house-cleaning. It will expel accumulated toxic wastes and morbid matters. It will free burdened organs so they can function normally again. The body corrects itself when the causes of its problems are removed." after DR. HERBERT SHELTON in FASTING CAN SAVE YOUR LIFE.

"How is a person who is already sick to be made less sick by swallowing or receiving a drug, medicine or pharmaceutical concoction that would make ill a person in good health? A sick person must not only overcome his affliction but also the drug poisons administered to him. This is, indeed, double jeopardy. What a healthy individual requires to maintain health, a sick person needs to regain it!" after DR. VIRGINIA VETRANO in NATURAL HYGIENE—MAN'S PRISTINE WAY OF LIFE.

The body is a whole unit and in sickness or in good health we must have a well balanced supply of our vital needs. The blind lead the blind down through the ages with excesses and over-concentration on one supposed 'cure-all.' Let us refer again to Shelton to give us a boost along the way. He says, 'Do not become one sided in your manner of living. You cannot remain or become well and strong through exercise alone, or through diet alone, or rest and sleep alone. Fresh air and sunshine alone are not enough. Do not imagine that by breathing alone, you can reach the heights. All these things are good, but life is more than exercise, or food and drink; more than thought or rest

and sleep. It is all these and more. Life must be lived as a whole.'
Jack Dunn Trop, in YOU DON'T HAVE TO BE SICK.

Why This Volume Had To Be Written

Americans must be made aware of the suffering and early death they unknowingly bring upon themselves. They must be taught how to achieve a high state of health. They must realize that their well-being in itself is the loftiest of causes and that they can pursue no nobler purpose in life than to seek well-being. They must be inspired to launch and diligently follow a health program that will bring them the fruits of wonderful health that the human biological heritage makes easily possible.

Americans must be made aware that ignorance in itself is not their obstacle but that they know so much—so much that is not true!

This volume is intended to supply the understanding, the knowledge and the practical methods whereby dynamic health can be achieved. It is hoped that this publication can likewise inspire YOU to cultivate the causes of good health, to reject the causes of disease and to dedicate yourself to helping others learn the simple truths about health.

As you are undoubtedly aware many people are stubborn and cling to their erroneous concepts, their bad habits and injurious practices in the face of all reason. Some even hold tenaciously to killing habits with the knowledge they are doing so! Life is not precious to them. This attiude alone is life defeating.

This speaks not of spineless creatures so much as it speaks of a sick society, of humans in the aggregate who are so pérverted, so depraved and so degenerated that there is seemingly, no hope for them.

Yet I am not convinced the case for America is hopeless. It is better to try in vain than not to try at all. I am persuaded that the majority of Americans would wholeheartedly embrace the valid health practices of NATURAL HYGIENE if they could be induced TO THINK, ever so little, FOR THEMSELVES! I feel that, if they could see the problem, THE TRUE STATE OF THINGS, and the simple solutions, they would awake from their lethargy and adopt the proper courses in life.

The problem is a gigantic one! I know that YOU will do what you can to help when you realize its seriousness. Every conscientious individual who sees the grievous wrongs in America is bound to devote some of his energies and resources to helping correct them.

ARE AMERICANS REALLY A HEALTHY PEOPLE?

Good Health in America is a downright myth! Contrary to what the medical profession, the press, radio and TV, in fact, our commercial masters would have us believe, health in America is in a woeful state. We realize less than half our true life potential, and much of our shortened lives is plagued with life sapping economic insecurity, chronic disease, tormenting hopes and general suffering.

Lest you underestimate the gravity of the problem or the extent of suffering and ruinous practices in America consider these unpleasant facts:

1. The U.S. Public Health Service recognizes a mere 3,000,000 of our over 210,000,000 population as being healthy! This is about 1½%!

2. 54% of all Americans die of heart disease! Over 50 million Americans suffer from severe heart disease. Autopsies of our most fit young men who died on the Korean battlefields showed that 77% of them already had heart disease! Biologists state that a healthy heart should serve the human organism for at least 300 years!

3. About one billion visits are made to physicians annually in the U.S.A.!

4. About 4,500,000 people each year are poisoned so seriously by their physicians as to require hospitalization! Tens of thousands die! The so-called side effects or adverse reactions of drugs is perfumed language for POISON EFFECTS! All drugs or "medicines" are inherently poisonous!

5. The U.S. ranks 89th among nations in death rate!

6. One out of every four Americans will have cancer! Cancer is the number one cause of

death of our children! WHY? There are some countries where almost no cancer exists.

7. Arthritis and rheumatic complaints will affect 77% of our adult population!

8. About 40,000,000 Americans suffer allergies!

9. 60% of the population suffer defective vision!

10. Over 79,000,000 Americans are obese, far more than half of Americans are overweight, yet nearly all Americans are malnourished in one way or another despite gross overeating!

11. 103,000,000 Americans (49%) suffer from AT LEAST ONE chronic disease or disability!

12. Over 30,000,000 Americans will spend sometime in a hospital each year!

13. 50% of Americans suffer from digestive disorders.

14. An estimated 25,000,000 Americans suffer from high blood pressure.

15. Over 7,000,000 children are mentally retarded, disturbed or otherwise seriously handicapped.

16. 98.5% of our population have bad teeth! 31,000,000 have no teeth of their own! Fillings, dental cavities, decayed and deformed teeth are so prevalent that they are considered normal! The average American child has six cavities by school age! Good teeth have the possibility to serve the human organism for several centuries without breakdown!

17. Over 20,000,000 Americans suffer from mental illness!

18. Life expectancy of a one-year-old is no more today than it was in 1900. Life expectancy is actually decreasing in the U.S.A.! Scientific studies indicate that a one-year-old can expect to live no longer than our ancestors did 10,000 years ago!

19. 58.6% of America's children cannot pass a physical fitness test!

20. Over 50,000,000 aspirins are taken daily in the U.S.A. This amounts to about 20,000,000 pounds of aspirin yearly! What a king-sized headache America suffers!

21. Nearly all Americans (almost 100%) suffer from digestive leukocytosis and a pathologically high heartbeat. These conditions are largely the results of a pathogenic diet, drug habits and lack of healthful practices.

22. Over 200,000,000 Americans are hooked on one or more drug habits! The drugs of most frequent use are caffeine, nicotinc, alcohol, salt, aspirin, theine, theobromine and vinegar.

23. Nearly 100% of American women suffer debilitating leukorrhea and its consequent monthly hemorrhaging. Unfortunately this disease is regarded as normal in women of child-bearing age.

24. Over 3,000,000,000 (that's three billion) sleeping pills are consumed annually. An estimated 13,000,000,000 barbiturate and amphetamine pills are ingested annually! Tranquilizers are a way of life!

25. Nearly 20,000,000 Americans submit to the surgeon's knife each year!

26. Murders, suicides, juvenile delinquency, narcotic addiction and other forms of crime are rife and increasing! A sick people make a sick nation.

I could give you a seemingly endless resume of such statistics but why go on? The National Center for Health Statistics of the U.S. Public Health Service publishes volumes that reflect the widespread pathology of Americans.

Tell me, does this describe a healthy or a happy nation?

I hope that you're convinced that good health in America is a myth, that matters are in a terrible state and that something constructive MUST BE DONE!

It is because of this that I felt compelled to prepare this volume for publication. So ominous are the problems that beset America that I ask you to adopt a sane program of health practices as advocated herein. It is with a deep sense of purpose and commitment that I urge you to do what you can to help the Society spread and perpetuate its program for bringing good health to America! There is much you can do as you'll learn.

America's Desperate Need For A Valid Health System

The medical system is an outright failure! For some 2,500 years it has been trying to give man dispensation for his health transgressions without success. It has been trying to salvage him from disease through medication (drugs) while man continued to indulge the injurious practices that resulted in disease.

Today there is a veritable army of medical practitioners and a far larger corps of support personnel. They have an arsenal of drugs, potions, pills, medicines, vaccines, serums, antibiotics and "miracle" treatments. They constantly seek new and "better" remedies, for, in all this time, they have not succeeded in vanquishing A SINGLE DISEASE, though they take credit for conquering many!

Despite all the "miracle" drugs and "scientific" discoveries, they are faced with a growing army of the diseased. Hospitals are built in ever increasing proliferation. Physicians are being trained by the thousands. Nursing candidates are being assured of employment even before their training begins. ARE WE DESTINED TO BECOME A NATION OF SICK PEOPLE?

Why does the multitude of the suffering continue to grow? Why do their illnesses become ever more complicated? Why are such disabling diseases as cancer and arthritis on the upsurge? Why do more and more of our people die of cancer and heart disease?

IS THE DETERIORATING HEALTH OF AMERICA A TESTIMONIAL TO THE VALIDITY OR TO THE INVALIDITY OF THE MEDICAL SYSTEM? Will you think about that for a moment?

For 2,500 years the highest powers of the human mind have been devoted to the invention or discovery of cures for the diseases of man. Many of the brightest minds have engaged in this search. Untold mountains of wealth have been poured into the effort to find cures.

For the past fifty years, "scientists" have devoted so much time, energy, talent and technical knowledge to this search that it makes all preceding efforts in this direction pale into insignificance. The whole field of nature has been ransacked to discover antidotes for the many diseases with which man suffers.

The chemist has analyzed every substance of nature, both organic and inorganic. He has created combinations as varied and numberless as the leaves of the forest. Not a mineral or a vegetable poison, however virulent, has escaped being tried or added to the truly frightful load of medicines to be used to cure man's diseases. The poisons of insects, of spiders, of snakes, as well as the execretions and puses of animals have been added to the materia medica. Can any sane person believe these are the elements of health?

In the hope of discovering some panacea or some specific for the ills of man, ambitious men have added thousands of drugs, or poisons, to the armanentarium of physicians.

Fortunes of tremendous magnitude have been acquired by the compounders of elixirs and cordials. Specifics galore have been announced with much hullabaloo. They have been tried and then gone their way—to give rise to new drugs. The results of all this searching and experimenting have not been fruitful. The search is now more feverish than ever! Ever greater expenditures are made. Yet diseases have increased; their malignancy and fatality have become more fearful. Chronic diseases, in particular, have enormously increased in modern times.

There are in this country more than 360,000 physicians; there are thousands upon thousands of hospitals, clinics, sanitoria; there are many giant chemical industries turning out drugs and vaccines; there are thousands of wholesale and retail drug companies, employing an army of pharmacists; there is a great army of nurses, technicians and others who depend on the drug trade for their livelihood. In addition to all these, there are the manufacturers of bottles, pill boxes, cartons and plastics, and there are the newspapers, magazines, radio and television that derive millions out of advertising these pernicious products. The drug industry, directly and indirectly, accounts for incomes and profits that run into many billions of dollars a year in this country alone. Yet, we are poverty stricken when it comes to good health!

Pitted against the bleak picture of disease that afflicts humanity is the greatest health discovery of all time—NATURAL HYGIENE—a way of living based on natural principles that enables human beings to remain in good health throughout life, and to return to good health in all remediable cases, if they are ailing.

The great, simple and most sublime truth which NATURAL HYGIENE reveals is that, incorporated in every living organism itself is a great vital regenerative capacity as part and parcel of its very life, identical with, and inseparable from, its very existence, by which and through which the organism developed. This vital power of the organism will, if not interfered with, always tend to keep the body in high functioning order—dynamic health! If an organism is diseased it will, permitted the opportunity, eliminate body wastes and accumulated morbid matters, repair and knit injuries, remove infirmities and heal its impairments.

The foes of NATURAL HYGIENE (usually those who have a vested interest in disease!) have been unable to demolish a single one of its basic principles or to discredit a single one of its essential practices, but, on the contrary, have strengthened it by all their genuine discoveries!

Every advance of knowledge in biology and

physiology has served to prove and confirm the scientific soundness of NATURAL HYGIENE and to remove the props from under the ancient practices of the medicine men.

Considering the vast importance of this body of truths and practices known as NATURAL HYGIENE and its role in both restoring and preserving health it would seem that it would be more widely appreciated and cultivated. It is to this task that the Society applies itself and for which it asks your aid.

The facts of NATURAL HYGIENE are so incontrovertible, however, that eventually the most incredulous will be compelled to accept them. The strongest prejudice must ultimately give way before the crushing reality of HYGIENIC truth.

The Essence of Natural Hygiene

A statement of NATURAL HYGIENE philosophy, principles and practice.

NATURAL HYGIENE is simple of principle and easily understood. It can be readily applied in life.

Once you have a steadfast grasp of its principles and understand how they appertain to life, you'll derive more benefit from it than from the mastery of all the intricate data and details science has discovered.

The principles of NATURAL HYGIENE, thoroughly proven in practice, are relatively new. This great health discovery was made early in the 19th Century. It was called HYGIENE, the science of health.

This new philosophy of health has as its basic tenets the following:

1. Vigorous robust health is the NORMAL STATE of human existence and, therefore, is realizable without interruption throughout life.

2. All physical maladies represent an ABNORMAL bodily state and, as such, are unnecessary and will not occur if we reject factors and influences not normal to the body and indulge those that are.

3. Only in nature which developed us to such

a high state can be found the solutions to the mysteries of disease, suffering and early death.

4. Therefore, only by living life in accord with man's particular adaptive experience as a creature of nature can he hope to achieve his high potential for health and happiness.

NATURAL HYGIENE emphasizes as the ESSENTIAL FACTORS of life and well-being those elements and influences which we adopted and adapted to during the course of our development in the lap of nature for millions of years.

These essential factors of life are as follows and are not necessarily enumerated in their order of vital importance:

1. PURE AIR
2. PURE WATER
3. CLEANLINESS
4. WARMTH
5. SLEEP
6. WHOLESOME FOOD
7. EXERCISE
8. REST AND RELAXATION
9. SUNSHINE
10. EMOTIONAL POISE.
11. PLEASANT ENVIRONMENT
12. SECURITY OF LIFE AND ITS MEANS
13. SELF-MASTERY
14. MOTIVATION
15. CREATIVE USEFUL WORK
16. BELONGING

17. EXPRESSION OF NATURAL INSTINCTS
18. INDULGENCE OF AESTHETIC SENSES

NATURAL HYGIENE teaches that the deficiency of these factors and influences, or any interference with their normal relationship to the organism is necessarily detrimental to human well-being.

NATURAL HYGIENE bases itself upon the recognition of these fundamental natural principles as they pertain to human health:

A. The human body, supplied with its physiological needs, is a self-sufficient organism with inherent powers capable of maintaining itself in good functioning order for the duration of its life potential, that is, from 120 or more years.

B. That all diseases or bodily malfunctions are caused by bodily abuse or by incorrect living, that is, failure to live in accord with and indulge the essential requirements of life as heretofore listed.

C. That, in the event of sickness or disease, (and a hygienist should have no such event) the body needs only the removal of or non-indulgence of cause or causes of malfunction to restore itself to health. That is to say that the body, conditions permitting, is SELF CORRECTING or SELF HEALING!

D. That body requirements in illness are the same as those when in a state of health except that a malfunctioning body requires complete physiological rest so that the body's restorative capabilities, that is, its regenerative and healing powers, may function fully and unhampered.

NATURAL HYGIENE finds that diseases are systemic malfunctions begotten by incorrect living that involves one or more of these inimical factors:

1. Improper eating, that is, eating the wrong foods; eating the correct foods in an unnatural state, which is to say, cooked, preserved or processed; eating foods in unphysiological combinations or overeating.

2. Insufficient sleep and/or rest.

3. Lack of fresh air.

4. Ingestion of toxic substances, either toxic in themselves, or as a part of our food and water intake.

5. Lack of exercise.

6. Lack of sunshine.

7. Over indulgence of normally harmless pursuits.

8. Indulgence of injurious habits.

9. Subjection to situations of emotional insecurity or emotional stress.

NATURAL HYGIENE teaches that all disease stems from NERVOUS EXHAUSTION, that is, the exhaustion of nerve energy or vital force. When the body's fund of nerve energy is overdrawn or undersupplied the body can no longer properly conduct vital functions efficiently or effectively.

When functional power is lowered the body's ability to eliminate metabolic wastes and unwelcome extraneous materials is hampered or, to illustrate graphically, we might say these morbid matters become dammed up in the system. The body is no longer equal to the task of expulsion of normal or abnormal wastes.

When unwelcome substances remain in the body the integrity of the body economy is threatened. The toxic load of unexpelled morbid wastes causes the body to resort to an emergency crisis to rid itself of a condition called toxemia or, very simply, toxic overload.

The emergency crisis to preserve bodily integrity through extraordinary cleansing efforts is exhibited as symptoms known as sickness, disease, illness, ailment, affliction or malady. In this abnormal state the small fund or remaining nerve energy is mustered to the task of body purification. Normal and emergency outlets for elimination of toxic matters are utilized. The form these crises of elimination take is labelled by their location and characteristics. Their characteristics or symptoms are called variously colds, fevers, inflammations, catarrhs or a long list of maladies ad nauseam—some 20,000 names of maladies have been catalogued. To hygienists all these crises, regardless of symptoms and characteristics, excepting those involving organic degeneration, are, pure and simple, toxemia. The body is loaded with more poisonous matters than it can tolerate in its current state of vitality.

When the body has completed the task of purification; when the body has purged itself of its toxic overload; when the accumulation of noxious matters have been reduced to a level commensurate with functioning in the current state of vitality, the subject is said to be healed or is well again.

Hygienists have formulated a system of health recognizing man's complete dependence upon nature and, therefore, the role of natural means in keeping us in a state of health and its agency in speedily restoring health if it is lost through our failure to live properly.

We can aid nature best in restoring health, in the event of its loss, by regeneration of our fund of nerve energy. This is best accomplished by not expending the small fund of nerve energy that remains but, instead, undertaking a physiological rest, A COMPLETE REST! This is known as a fast. A fast is the complete abstinence from all food except the only three inorganic nutrients man is capable of utilizing, that is, pure water, fresh air and sunshine.

NATURAL HYGIENE implores us to heed our natural requirements for well-being and to indulge them prudently and wisely. This constitutes the science of correct living.

An Elaboration Upon Eighteen Factors and Influences Essential To Superb Health and Well-Being

The eighteen factors and influences listed here are not necessarily an exhaustive list. Neither are they free of redundancy for some factors imply the others. Further, listing in an order of importance is somewhat meaningless for most of these factors are as important as the other though all may not have the same immediacy to vital existence.

I cannot emphasize too strongly that a judicious adherence to the needs of well-being will assure the follower, if his constitution is sound and he suffers no previously contracted organic impairments, a life of at least 120 to 160 years completely FREE of diseases, ailments, maladies, derangements, impairments, debilities or what have you.

These factors and influences are elaborated as follows:

1. PURE AIR. Pure air is free of pollutants of all kinds with only the "normal" amount of carbon dioxide, carbon monoxide, inert gases

and particulates which the body is well equipped to handle. Man has adapted to these over millions of years. Unfortunately, air today is loaded with immense amounts of these substances plus numerous other pollutants and outright poisons. Today we get only a fraction of the oxygen rich fresh air we need and are wont to stay in homes and work places where we constantly inhale our own aerial excreta and staggering amounts of pollutants into our lungs. Further, most Americans burden their lungs with pollutants of the worst nature in smoking —it is a deadly poison habit—a narcotic addiction that slowly kills. Make it a practice to get as much fresh air as your circumstances will permit. The ideal is to live in completely fresh air such as it is in a pristine state of nature! If all other circumstances were equal, scientists say that living only in fresh air would increase life expectancy considerably.

2. PURE WATER. The water ingested by humans must be, ideally, completely free of impurities, that is, chemicals, inorganic minerals and other substances. Only distilled water adequately fulfills this requirement, but as man is not a drinking animal except in abnormal situations, pure water requirements can be met from a water sufficient diet of fruits, vegetables and nuts. Almost all water drinking in present day Americans is pathological. Except in rare situations, hygienists do not experience thirst. Water drinking animals either lap water with their tongue or have elongated heads so formed

that they can draw water with facility by suction. Man is not a drinking animal and his cousins in nature, the anthropoids, live on water sufficient diets of fruits, vegetables and nuts as, indeed, do many desert animals that do not drink water in their whole lifetime.

Hard or mineralized waters should be shunned for they are all harmful to the human economy. The human body cannot utilize any mineral as found in water NO MATTER HOW IMPORTANT these very same minerals are to our bodies!

We need iron but would you think of eating iron filings? We need calcium but can you conceive of eating powdered lime? We need magnesium but would you grind up a smidget of it and consume it? Water leaches minerals from the soil and rocks through which it passes but the mineral held in solution is of no more use to the human body than if it were eaten in soil form.

If the human body could utilize minerals in inorganic form there would be no objection in eating soil or, better yet, drinking sea water! In fact, sea water would be best of all as it contains ALL minerals man requires! But there is an objection—the objection of the human body itself! Drink a glass of sea water and the body will speedily eject it!

No mineral, or compound of it, can be utilized by the body EXCEPT in colloidal form as compounded organically BY PLANT LIFE! Otherwise, minerals are just so much more noxious matter in the system. Anything taken into the body that is not utilizable is a poison. The body treats inorganic minerals as found in water as poisons and expels them from the system as best it can. Uneliminated inorganic minerals are "tucked away" in the system where they will do the least harm but they collect and collect and eventually give us harmful deposits just as they do in clogging water pipes, tea kettles, etc.

Ill health begets more ill health. If the body is in an impaired state, it cannot eliminate mineral or other wastes as it should. Inorganic minerals are some of the raw materials of stones that form in the body, hardening of the arteries, ossifying of the brain, etc. As water drinking is largely pathological in the first place it is an impaired organism that drinks and furthers its pathology.

Fruits and vegetables can be a water-sufficient diet ONLY if uncooked! Cooked foods are pathogenic! Abnormal amounts of water are required to "flush" out or carry out the noxious matters created in food by cooking. I have seen people eat highly liquid soup with its spices, seasonings and salt and develop a fierce thirst as a result! This is some indication of just how pathogenic a diet of cooked and seasoned foods are.

If you must drink, and you should drink when the body demands water through thirst, drink DISTILLED WATER! All other waters are to be avoided. Remember, drink ONLY when thirsty and drink only distilled water,

Never drink when not thirsty. Your body is a reliable guide as to its water requirements and has the mechanisms to make you aware of its needs.

3. CLEANLINESS, INTERNAL AND EXTERNAL. Almost all Americans pursue a program of external cleanliness that is adequate insofar as it keeps our skin clean. In fact, it goes too far! It goes so far as to be, actually, injurious!

We bathe ourselves daily to free ourselves of skin excreta and unwelcome substances that may come onto the skin. Only water should be used in cleansing and a flesh brush. We should abjure such harmful substances as soaps, powders, shampoos, cosmetics, toothpastes, bracers etc. External cleansing is a *MECHANICAL, NOT* a CHEMICAL process! But daily bathing is wise and desirable because an accumulation of substances on the skin bring into play our friendly scavengers, bacteria. Unfortunately, the end-products of bacterial activity are more poisonous to us than our own toxic excreta, as a rule.

Internal cleanliness means the *COMPLETE* elimination of noxious matters that the body generates as a result of metabolism and which may be taken into the body unintentionally or, perhaps, intentionally.

Cleanliness, or body purification, is a continuous body function and occurs 100% of our lives. The cleansing process varies in intensity according to our daily biological clock. In most humans it is most pronounced between 3:00 A.M. and 7:00 A.M.

There are four primary organs that are points of elimination. Our lungs are our primary organ of elimination. Our skin, kidneys and bowels are the other points of elimination in roughly their order of vital importance. The mucous membranes, while still skin, internal skin that is, are compensatory organs of elimination. The liver is an organ of elimination but is not an exit point for morbid matters. In emergencies the body may utilize the organs less essential to the body economy as points of accumulation of toxic garbage. When such occurs we have inflamed organs such as in tonsilitis or appendicitis.

There is much we can do to insure internal cleanliness. First, of course, is to live healthfully in accord with the dictates of our natural endowment. We should utilize non-toxic foods that are "clean burning" in the digestive and assimilative processes and furnish the broadest range of nutrients the body requires. To assure rather thorough internal cleanliness our regimen for living should include regular fasting, exercise, sunbathing, adequate sleep, pure water, pure air, etc., in fact, the very factors and influences we are now discussing.

4. SLEEP. The body can more efficiently conduct certain of its daily "restocking activities", that is, the regeneration of nerve energy the assimilation and distribution of fuel and nutrients, the replacement of spent cells, etc. under

a condition that conserves the use of vital body nutrients and forces. This condition is the somnolent state which we call sleep. While in a state of sleep the body can concentrate its activities on assimilation of food ingested during the prior alimentary period, restocking the cells, the liver and other tissue and organs with fuel, regenerating nerve force, replacing spent cells and, as a night cap, it goes into an extraordinary "house cleaning" of accumulated food and metabolic debris. Sleep, as a daily restorative process, is one of our most essential functions. You can favor it by observing the optimum conditions for sound sleep. These are too involved to present in this small volume but the more salient are repose in a quiet serene surrounding with pure fresh air, a well ventilated body kept at a comfortable temperature on a bed as comfortable as we can obtain.

5. TEMPERATURE MAINTENANCE. The normal body temperature of a healthy individual is perhaps nearly a degree lower than the 98.6 established as "normal" by the medical profession. Increased temperature may be indicative of increased pathology. Keeping warm involves proper dress so that our bodies are clothed suitably for conserving our bodily heat if cold or for permitting maximum ventilation and cooling of the body if the atmosphere is unduly warm. Never shock the body with cold or hot temperatures such as experienced from cold air or water or from hot air or water. Wear clothing that permits the maximum

ventilation while yet permitting retention of needed body heat. Generally this will mean the rejection of synthetic fibres as clothing and the use of cotton goods.

6. PURE WHOLESOME FOOD. On this subject almost all "health conscious" persons are concerned to the near exclusion of the other factors that weigh vitally upon health. And it is here that I find the most controversy. Admittedly our aliment is the predominant factor weighing upon the condition of our health. Some assess food as being 75% of the game of health. I would not rate it this high but I would not rate it below 50% as an essential factor for well-being for the physiological basis for optimum health lies primarily in the wholesomeness of our diet.

Food must be, ideally, free of contaminants, chemicals, additives, preservatives, inorganic minerals and even harmful substances that are natural to some of them. The body has great capacity for handling and expelling unwelcome substances but it is a capacity wisely not put to use. The roughages of foods have not been determined to be essential to nutrition but are necessary to our well-being for our digestive systems have come to be dependent upon foods containing roughages.

The aliments worthy of human nourishment are: A. FOODS *NATURAL* to man's dietary as established by millions of years of eating and digestive adaptation, B. *FOOD NURTURED* by *NATURAL* means, that is foods that contain their natural constituents by virtue of being raised strictly by natural means and supplied with their nutrient requirements, C. FOODS *SERVED* in their *NATURAL STATE*, that is, in the condition in which nature delivers them to us, untampered with in any way and D. ingested in a manner and combination compatible to our physiological capability of digesting and making use of them. The only foods that ideally serve man's total requirements are *LIVING FOODS* with their enzymes, auxones, hormones, vitamins, minerals, proteins, fats and carbohydrates INTACT, alive and untampered with. This means we'll eat foods that are not in any way cooked or preserved. It means we'll eat only foods that are a gustatory delight in their pristine state such as are most fruits, nuts and vegetables.

If we eat foods natural to the palate and body economy of man in the fashion outlined, our diet is bound to be about 90% alkaline. A predominantly alkaline diet is essential to our wellbeing.

Man's natural foods are fruits, nuts and succulent green leaves. Ideally his dietary admits of little else. As most disease evolves from dietary transgressions our sole objective with respect to food should be to eat those most suited for our optimal health.

7. EXERCISE. For ideal health daily exercise is very essential. All muscles of the body, over 700 of them, should be activated in some manner every day. Unused muscles atrophy.

Muscles put to daily activity develop and serve us. They make us feel alive and give us a certain eagerness to do things.

Most exercise and physical work tends to ignore the muscles of the eyes, neck, head, ears, stomach, etc. A varied exercise program is good but indulgence in meaningful and purposeful physical activities such as gardening and its varied chores is much better for us. Creative work should involve physical activity where possible. Recreational sports are especially good. This involves running, non-contact sports, skating, etc. Indolence and inactivity are the enemies of our well-being. If you would have perpetual health and happiness indulge in vigorous physical activity, even strenuous physical activity, for some part of each day. Of course if you have not exercised for "ages" you should begin your exercise program on a gradual but increasing basis for vigorous and strenuous exercise can be deadly to atrophied bodies.

8. SUNSHINE. This is an elusive factor for most northerners for a part of the year. The ideal is to obtain a few minutes of sunshine every day up to about 30 minutes. It is absolutely essential to optimum health. It is a vital factor in the body's synthesis of the vital nutrient called Vitamin D. While sunflower seeds and sea vegetation contain some Vitamin D there is no real substitute for the beneficial rays of the sun upon the body. Even in Northern climes it is possible to get the benefits of sunshine a few days each month, even during the

coldest periods except, of course, in the farthest North. Getting sunshine in the coldest months will depend to a great extent on how ingenious we are or how well we can manage it when the sun is out.

9. REST AND RELAXATION. The body should be relieved of tension and tension-creating situations as may be "normal" to your role in present day society. Two or three times daily we should just relax, let go and get our minds off problems which may oppress us. A nap is often a great regenerator of our vital powers, even a simple nap of a few minutes. We should relax for about 20 to 30 minutes before meals until we have slowed our "engines" down. Further, we should relax after meals for part of the blood is then occupied with the digestive processes and should not be drawn to other activity lest we suffer impaired digestion. Sleep is supreme as a form of rest and recuperator of our vital powers. We should get ample sleep and intersperse our day with brief periods of rest and relaxation if we would have the best health.

10. EMOTIONAL POISE. This is a state wherein we always feel well, secure and socially worthwhile. Feeling well is the result of the foregoing cited factors and those cited hereafter. Our emotional state is dictated by our physiological state and our environmental influences. Strive for the best of both as, indeed, this is an outline of the necessity to achieve the best of both.

11. SECURITY OF LIFE AND ITS

MEANS. Everyone is best emotionally and, therefore, physically if he not only has the wherewithal of life, but he is in an "unthreatened" situation with assurance of his life and those he concerns himself with and, further, that the necessities and reasonable wants of life will be available upon reasonable effort. Moreover, man is in a state of emotional equilibrium or happy when he is satisfied that he has received the full social value of the labor he has expended in the productive process and only a society in which such a condition exists will see man achieve his true health potential.

12. PLEASANT ENVIRONMENT. This concerns our total surroundings including not only our domestic situation as it involves our family, home and grounds but our geographical surroundings, climate, our work conditions, the people in our lives, society at large, the "territory" we frequent etc. We should always strive to have an environment that makes us feel at ease and contented.

13. CREATIVE USEFUL WORK. We should always involve ourselves in activity productive of useful products and services that meet both our and society's needs. If we involve ourself in "dead" or "parasitical" pursuits our disposition will reflect the unwholesomeness of our occupation. Our health tends to be likewise impaired. Only socially useful work should be engaged in and, preferably, work that challenges our intellectual faculties. We should avoid dull, repetitive and uncreative pursuits.

We should have hobbies that also involve us in the betterment of ourselves and our society. I suggest gardening as one of the most wholesome of hobbies.

14. SELF-MASTERY. Self discipline, self-control, a general awareness of ourselves and our environment with a confident and intelligently guided response to that which involves us comprises self-mastery. Unknown to most people are the joys of mastering themselves in situations where they would ordinarily act unthinkingly or act out of sheer impulse or appetancy.

15. BELONGING. Man is a gregarious creature and he can live healthier in association with others of similar disposition. Being accepted by a group or a social circle that has captivated our fealty is a most wholesome influence emotionally.

16. MOTIVATION. The happiest and healthiest individuals are those who have innate drives to achieve objectives they recognize as worthy. Motivation means dedication, purpose, direction, intent and ambition to achieve socially meritorious ends.

17. EXPRESSION OF THE NATURAL INSTINCTS. While the foregoing largely cover the instincts we cannot omit the expression of a very basic instinct to perpetuate the species, that is, the reproductive instinct. While our innate sexuality should be indulged it is, in our society, all too often a morbid matter pursued

as an end in itself. It is an escapist outlet to release pentup emotions that should not occur in the first place. Basically, the instinct of reproduction is for one purpose only, the perpetuation of the species. But nature has been lavish and has bestowed upon us sexual urge in excess of actual need to insure the survival of the species. Expression of this instinct in keeping with our physiological capabilities and limitations is of beneficence to our well-being.

18. INDULGENCE OF THE AESTHETIC SENSES. The human ability to appreciate beauty, art and goodness is not unique but it is so highly developed as to place us far above the most advanced animals. To achieve optimum health we should be surrounded by the beauty in nature and in man's art. We should be in association with those whose lives, personalities, attitudes and deportment are pleasing to our social senses. Unaesthetic surroundings, people of ugly disposition and a paucity of beauty influences deeply and tends to likewise shape individuals.

The needs of life are this simple! Nothing is complicated about it. It seems self-evident that these are the essential means for a happy and healthy life. We can see that the science of health does not come from the so-called scientific laboratories but, instead, it springs from the laboratory of nature. Hygienists maintain that this comprises the basic formula by which man lived in the lap of nature while developing into the superb creature that he really is. Perhaps we can pursue no wiser course than to cultivate optimally these factors and influences in our pattern of living.

What Is Natural Hygiene?

NATURAL HYGIENE is a way of life that allows those with health to keep it . . . . those who have lost health to regain it . . . and those who never have had health to experience it.

NATURAL HYGIENE defines good health as having the most strength and endurance that one can build, as "feeling good" all the time, as being efficient and useful throughout a long and happy life.

The practice of NATURAL HYGIENE includes a balance of those things usually included in any conventional health program, such as fresh air, pure water, sunshine, sleep, exercise, relaxation, and mental and emotional poise.

However, NATURAL HYGIENE departs from the conventional by advocating (1) A diet made up exclusively of fruits, nuts and green leafy vegetables, organically grown and eaten raw. (2) Rejecting as harmful all medicines, treatments and cures customarily employed in dealing with illness. (3) Suggesting fasting (total abstinence from all food except water) as a proper practice when well (if desired) and as an essential practice in (most) sickness and disease.

NATURAL HYGIENE bases its position in regard to diet on two principles: (1) Man is

acknowledged to be the highest form of animal life. In terms of his physical body man belongs to a group of animals known as primates which includes monkeys, chimpanzees and gorillas. These animals, as they become more man-like in appearance, tend to live more exclusively on fruits, nuts and green leafy vegetables, and less on other foods. Man also is in a class known as the mammals who are warm-blooded, hair-covered, live-bearing, milk-producing animals, and eat special foods in keeping with their make up. Dogs, cats and lions are meat eaters. Cows, horses, sheep, deer, camels and goats are grain, grass and cereal eaters. Pigs and other swine are scavengers and eat almost anything.
(2) Cooking and processing destroy and degrade nutritional values in foods.

NATURAL HYGIENE denies that germs and viruses cause disease. It declares that man builds disease through wrong living. This includes improper eating, inactivity and over-activity, over-stimulation and other forms of indulgences which raise the body's toxicity level while lowering its fund of vital nerve energy.

NATURAL HYGIENE abhors any indulgence in tobacco, alcohol, coffee, tea, drugs, narcotics and all other physiological and psychological practices disturbing and detrimental to life and health. It likewise abhors over-indulgence (gluttony) in those practices usually considered normal and essential to life and health. Prime examples are overeating, over-exposure to sun and sexual excess.

NATURAL HYGIENE rejects the use of drugs, medicines, inoculations, vaccines, x-rays, blood transfusions, vitamin pills, food supplements, and all other "treatments" as being of any use in restoring the body to a state of health. NATURAL HYGIENE views these things as interfering and harmful to life and health.

As alternatives NATURAL HYGIENE offers supervised bed rest and fasting in a calm, quiet environment as the most effective, efficient sensible means of dealing with (most) illness and disease.

It is obvious and provable that healing (getting well) is a normal activity of the body. When you burn, bruise or cut yourself or when a surgeon operates or sets a broken bone, it is the body that heals itself, not the salve, bandage, merthiolate, stitches, cast nor the surgeon. Healing is a normal body process which goes on all the time in relation to the amount of energy available for it.

The body has only so much energy available to do all the things it has to do. The amount of energy consumed in physical movement each day is significant. The amount of energy used in eating, digesting, absorbing and assimilating food is tremendous. Bed rest and fasting allow the body to save all this energy and use it to repair tissue, restore function and "clean house" in general.

NATURAL HYGIENE is prepared to substantiate its premises and promises through logic, statistics, available research and experimentation and testimonials. However, NATURAL HYGIENE suggests that real proof for YOU can be had best by learning more about this unusual and rewarding way of life by living it. A short program of self experimentation, say for the next 30 days, will thrill and amaze you. It could change the course of your whole life. You might never be the same. Surely you will be richer, healthier and wiser for having investigated and tried "Nature's Way to Normal Living."

Fasting as a Part of Your Dynamic Health Program

Regular fasting of from one to three days will prove a great health boon! Your author abstains from all food from Sunday evenings until Tuesday noons and finds this weekly fasting period one of the most efficacious of health practices.

Without doubt Dr. Herbert M. Shelton is the world's greatest authority on fasting. He has supervised the fasts of more than 40,000 people. Understanding the heightened healing powers the body can exercise while fasting is essential if you are to practice the Hygienic Program. Therefore, it is most appropriate that we include here a chapter from Dr. Shelton's best selling book, FASTING CAN SAVE YOUR LIFE.—CHAPTER I—FASTING AND YOU.

Fasting is much more than simply not eating: it is both a science and an art. It has meaning in terms of overall well-being and affects the psychological and emotional aspects of our lives.

Fasting, as we use the term here, means total abstinence from all food for a definite period of time. The word comes from the old English word *faesten*, which means firm or fixed. In other words, the fast is something we hold to on a firm basis under controlled and fixed conditions.

In religious terms it may mean abstinence from certain food on certain holy days. But this is partial abstinence rather than total abstinence. I know persons who have "fasted" during Lent and actually gained weight rather than lost, because they substituted for the dishes they gave up foods which put on even more pounds.

Those who think that fasting is equivalent to starvation are entirely wrong. There are basically two periods in the process of abstaining from food that should concern us here—the *fasting* period proper and the period of *starvation*.

As we study the phenomena of abstinence in greater detail, the distinction between these two phases will become clear. From the outset however, it is essential to understand that the fasting stage continues so long as the body supports itself on the stored reserves within its tissues. Starvation begins when abstinence is carried beyond the time when these stored reserves are used up or have dropped to a dangerously low level.

We must understand also that there is much loose terminology that adds to confusion on the subject of fasting. For example: we hear people speak of going on a "water fast" which technically would imply that they were giving up drinking water. What they mean, actually, is that they are going on a fast in which they give up everything but water. The same illogicality exists in the expression, "going on a fruit juice fast" or a "vegetable juice fast." Again what is meant is that they are giving up everything *except* fruit or vegetable juice.

The term "partial fast" is used for any form of fasting where individuals put extremely limiting conditions on what they eat. The misuse of the word "*starving*," not only in the venacular, but even in some scientific papers, has done vast harm. The word is derived from the Anglo-Saxon *stearfan*, which means to die, not only from lack of food but also from overall exposure to cold. This is how the phrase "starving cold" developed.

Starvation is a process of dying, in effect. You cannot starve yourself into good health. You can fast for proper and reasonable periods and thereby improve your physical condition and often restore yourself to good health. It is possible to abstain from food for long periods of time with beneficial effects. At the point where the experienced advisor who conducts the fast realizes that the second phase of abstention from food is imminent, the fast is broken.

I have said the fast is part of a new way of life which I outline in this book. Thus it is not used only to lose weight. It can be and certainly is equally important as a part of the function of maintaining or even restoring good health.

The sick or wounded animal finds a secluded

spot where he can keep warm, where he is protected from the weather, where he can have peace and quiet and be undisturbed. There he rests and fasts. He may, for example, have lost a limb, but he lies there in his privacy and generally recovers without drugs, without bandages or surgery.

In the animal world fasting is a tremendously important factor of existence. Animals fast not only when sick or wounded but also during hibernation or aestivation (sleeping throughout the summer in tropical climates).

Some animals fast during the mating season and in many cases during the nursing period. Some birds fast while their eggs are being hatched. Some animals fast immediately after birth. There are forms of spiders who do not eat for six months after they are born. Some wild creatures fast when taken into captivity, and a domestic pet, a dog, or a cat, may not eat for several days when it comes into a new environment. Animals also survive forced fasts during periods of drought, snow, cold, and live for long periods when no food is available.

In mankind fasting has been practised in various parts of the world over centuries for religious reasons, for self-discipline, for political purposes and as a means of restoring health. Only in recent centuries has the concept that we must eat to keep up our strength become a deeply entrenched idea. Dr. Felix Oswald, a Dutch physician who came to America before the turn of the century, declares: "The fast cure method is not limited to our dumb fellow creatures. It is a common experience that pain, fever, gastric congestion and even mental afflictions take away the appetite and only unwise nurses will try to thwart the purposes of Nature in this respect."

Fasting is centuries old; we read of it in the Bible and in Homer. It was employed in the care of the sick in ancient temples in Egypt, Greece and throughout the Mediterranean world. The use of the fast in acute disease dates back to remote times.

It was prescribed by Arabian physicians during the long dark night of Europe's Medieval Age. In Italy, Neapolitan physicians as long ago as one hundred and fifty years, employed fasts that sometimes lasted for forty days in the case of fever patients.

This writer has been engaged in conducting fasts since the summer of 1920. In this period of approximately forty-five years, I have conducted thousands of fasts ranging from a few days duration to ninety days, both for weight reduction and in connection with helping the body recover from physical impairment.

One particular case of an elderly man is of special interest because the results were so successful.

Mr. A.B. was seventy years of age and had been sick a large part of those years. For thirteen years he had suffered with bronchial asthma and during this time he had been hospitalized five times. For an even longer time he had suffered with sinus trouble. For six years he had been completely deaf in his left ear, while he had suffered with an enlarged prostate gland for more than six years and had been impotent for a few years. He wore glasses, was bald headed, and had the usual "minor symptoms" that indicate the condition of his organism was not good, although it is common to ignore these evidences of incipient disease.

Although he had been treated by the usual methods over the years, he had realized no genuine benefits from this care. Like others who suffer as he did, he grew from bad to worse. It is generally known that the regular care of asthmatics is purely palliative and that the patient commonly grows progressively worse with the passage of time. It is equally well known that the regular modes of care fail to do more than provide doubtful temporary relief for the sufferer with sinus disease. It seems hardly necessary to add that nothing of real value is done for deafness and for enlargement of the prostate gland. All of these conditions are commonly understood to be *incurable*.

Leaving his hospital bed in Chicago, the fifth time he was hospitalized for asthma, Mr. A.B. went directly to the airport and boarded a plane going south and went to a place that was reputed to be very successful in its care of asthma sufferers. Still wheezing, he was uncertain that he could make the trip, but had determined to try. His own statement was that he had suffered enough and that he was convinced that the regular methods of care offered him no real promise of health. Like many thousands of other asthmatics, he had given the regular plans of care every opportunity to free him effectively of his suffering and they had failed him.

Arriving at the institution in the southwest, he was admitted and told that he would have to discontinue at once and thereafter all drugs that he had been using for relief. "But," he asked, "what shall I do if I have an attack of asthma?"

"You will grit your teeth and clench your fists and suffer through it," was the reply. "You cannot get well if you continue to use drugs."

He was sent to bed and instructed to remain there and take nothing into his mouth but water until he was told that he could resume eating. The treatment is going to be worse than the disease, he thought. Could he go without food? He was weak from years of suffering and from a lengthy period during which he was unable to secure enough oxygen. He was assured that he would be carefully watched and that no harm would befall him.

With a certain amount of trepidation he entered upon what was to be a new and surprisingly pleasant experience. Fasting is not always a pleasant experience, but it can be a very interesting and even highly pleasurable experience. The freedom and ease that one experiences during a period of abstinence from food often enables one to discover new and previously undreamed-of depths of meaning to life.

About four o'clock in the morning of his first night of fasting, Mr. A.B. developed a severe paroxysm of asthma. He was unable to breathe while lying in bed, so he sat up on the side of the bed and rang for assistance. The doctor came and after observing and examining him, said: "You'll be all right in a brief time. It will take about twenty-four hours for you to become free of asthmatic symptoms, and then you'll be comfortable."

When the doctor left, Mr. A.B. was struggling for air. "What kind of a place have I come to," Mr. A.B. asked the man in the next bed. "They won't even do anything to relieve me of my attack." He continued to struggle for air for a few more minutes, then relief came and he fell asleep.

When the doctor saw him again in the morning, Mr. A.B. was feeling so well that he was ready to forgive the seeming neglect of the latter part of the night. He was more than overjoyed when he went on day after day breathing as easily as when he was a small boy, with not the slightest sign of asthma. He had not another single paroxysm of asthma so long as he remained at the institution. His sinuses were still draining and the fast was continued. After about six days without food, he was able to void urine as freely as a boy. His prostate gland had shrunken to nearly normal size.

He continued to fast and watched a day by

day disappearance of symptoms, until his sinuses cleared up, his breathing was a pleasure and his chest was a source of real joy. On the twenty-fifth day of the fast, he asked the doctor if he could not break the fast. He was informed that this would be premature, that he was not fully recovered and that it would be wise to continue. "You are not in jail," said the doctor. "You cannot be made to fast against your will. But, if you want my best advice you will continue for a while."

He took the doctor's advice and went ahead with the fast. What will always seem to him as a miracle was the fact that on the thirty-sixth day of the fast, he regained his hearing in his deaf ear. His hearing was so good that he could easily hear the low ticking of a small watch when held at arm's length from his ear. Equally important is the fact that the recovery of hearing was permanent. The fast was continued through the forty-second day and then feeding was resumed.

But he had another surprise in store for him. He discovered, upon his return home, a few weeks after the fast was broken, that he was no longer impotent. As restoration of potency in men and overcoming of frigidity in women are not uncommon results of the fast, this was no surprise to the head of the institution.

This is no fanciful case, but an actual account of the recovery of a man who had suffered as I have described and who underwent the fast, as I have here portrayed it, and who made the recovery that has been pictured. It was not an unusual case, except in the variety of conditions that he suffered with, unless we say that the recovery of hearing is not a rule when the deaf undergo a fast. It is only an occasional result of fasting. This is so because deafness, like loss of vision, may be due to a variety of abnormal conditions of the ear, and not all of them are remediable. Blindness is only occasionally recoverable by fasting for the same reason, although restoration of good vision, in errors of refraction, is not at all uncommon.

The dramatic recoveries that occur during a fast of proper length and taken under the most favorable conditions can be believed only by those who have had opportunity to observe them. The general tendency of both the layman and the physician, when hearing stories of such recoveries, is to dismiss them as too fantastic for consideration. Yet, there is nothing miraculous about the effects of the fast. If we think on the matter a little, we cannot escape the conclusion that fasting is the most natural and the most sensible means of care of the sick body of which we have any knowledge.

For over one hundred and forty years, Natural *Hygienists* have employed the fast as a means of promoting health and enabling the body to recover speedily from illness. They have amassed extraordinary clinical experience in this area. These experiences turn into the deeply-rooted conviction that the fast is a constructive force which must be utilized and developed as part of the regular practices of modern life.

There are, of course, critics of fasting. Most of them know very little about fasting, or its techniques. A. Rabogliati, A.M., M.D., F.R.C.S., of England so well puts it: "The most popular criticisms of fasting are written by people who have never missed a meal in their lives."

Whether it is to maintain or to restore good health, to gain weight or to lose weight, the role of fasting is a vital factor that can no longer be overlooked by any who are concerned with personal health and well-being—mentally and physically.

How You Can Enjoy Superb Health

Your Daily
Program for Well-being

- NATURAL HYGIENE (THE HEALTHFUL WAY OF LIVING) CONSISTS OF MANY PARTS.
- ALL PARTS MUST BECOME INVOLVED IN YOUR DAILY LIFE.
- THIS TELLS YOU WHAT THESE PARTS ARE—HOW TO USE EACH PART—WHAT NOT TO DO THAT IS COMMONLY DONE AND IS HARMFUL.

FOOD

DO
- Eat only fruits, nuts and vegetables. (see list further along)
- Eat mostly uncooked food. An all living food diet is ideal.
- Learn the proper rules of food combining. ("Food Combining Made Easy" is a good reference on the subject.)
- Eat foods at room temperature.

- Chew thoroughly! Digestion begins in the mouth.
- Eat foods in their whole form, with skins on when edible, such as apples and pears, if organically grown.
- Make your meals look attractive.
- Avoid product that is wilted.
- Eat only when relaxed.
- Eat raw food before cooked food.
- Eat only when hungry.

DON'T
- Cook fruits or nuts.
- Cook with butter or fat of any kind.
- Overeat.
- Eat when in pain, emotionally upset, tired, or immediately after hard work.
- Fry, boil or bake. Steam only.
- Season your foods.
- Eat foods that are strong tasting, such as onions, garlic, radishes, watercress, parsley.

PHYSICAL ACTIVITY

DO
- Involve all parts of the body when exercising.
- Exercise vigorously enough to cause heavy breathing, unless contra indicated.
- Make vigorous use of muscles, preferably against resistance.
- Exercise in fresh air, or with windows open, when indoors.

DON'T
- Exercise to the point of exhaustion.

- Deep breathe without being active at the same time.
- Exercise immediately following a meal.
- Prolonged muscular contractions beyond a few seconds.

POSTURE

DO
- Sit erect at all times.
- Keep head straight up while standing, sitting or walking.
- Keep work or reading material toward you, instead of moving toward it, when engaged in sedentary activity.

REST

DO
- Cease activity sometime during the day by sitting or preferably lying down.
- Close the eyes.
- Shut out light in the room as well as sound, if possible.
- Rest when tired.
  (If you have only a few minutes to rest, it is of value. Ten minutes is better, and 30 minutes to an hour is best.)

DON'T
- Read or watch television while resting.

SLEEP

DO
- Go to bed early.

- Select a dark, quiet and well ventilated room.
- Maintain a comfortable temperature.
- Practice a few moments of mental and physical quiet before retiring.

DON'T
- Eat an extra meal before retiring.

AIR

DO
- Get as much fresh air as possible.
- Allow ventilation to maximum extent, when indoors.
- Walk on streets which have less vehicular traffic.
- Insure that indoor air is free from contaminants, such as sprays of all kinds and circulated dust, that sometimes occurs when vacuuming.

DON'T
- Breathe through your mouth.
- Breathe excessively cold air, if at all possible.
- Breathe tobacco smoke.
- Permit smoking in your home, or in a private office if you have one.

TEMPERATURE

DO
- Maintain a comfortable temperature at all times.
- Dress for comfort and not for fashion.

DON'T
- Take hot or cold baths.

LIGHT AND SUNSHINE

DO
- Expose as much of your skin to light as possible. (Before dressing in the morning is a good time.)
- Use natural and not artificial light.
- Get the sun directly on your skin.
  (The rays penetrate only white, porous clothing.)
- Use an enclosure to cut off the wind, in inclement weather.
- Get your sun in cold climates through an open window while indoors, with artificial heat turned on to avoid undue chilling.
- Get all the sun possible daily up to an hour maximum, (preferably in the morning or afternoon).
- Get sun on the closed eyelids.

DON'T
- Remain in the sun for long periods.
  (This is a waste of nerve energy and dries the skin excessively)
- Expose yourself to the noonday sun.
- Use suntan lotion.
- Wear sunglasses.

WATER

DO
- Drink only when thirsty.

- Drink only enough to quench your thirst and no more.
- Drink distilled or soft water.

DON'T
- Drink with your meals

CLOTHING

DO
- Buy clothes of porous material.
- Wear light colored clothing.

DON'T
- Wear constricting clothing, such as girdles, tight belts, etc.

EXPRESSION OF THE EMOTIONS

DO
- Find something about which to be happy every day.
- Feed your emotions daily with good thoughts, pleasant sights and sounds, kind words, kindly touch, good deeds.
- Couple negative emotions, such as fear, grief, or anger, with physical activity.
- Keep negative emotions at a minimum.

ZEST FOR LIVING

DO
- Pursue some constructive objective.
- Engage in some activity which gives you fulfillment.

- Find a hobby which brings enjoyment, if your work is dissatisfying.

GENERAL

DON'T
- Take drugs or laxatives.
- Use vitamin pills and food supplements.

OBTAINING NUTRITIOUS FOOD

When so much of today's food is sprayed with poisonous chemicals, how may one insure a healthful food supply?

By growing your own sprouts!

Why are sprouts of value?

They are an excellent source of adequate protein that can be made fresh daily.

What kind of sprouts can one grow?

Mung bean, Alfalfa, Soy Beans, and other seeds.

Is it difficult to grow sprouts?

No, it is very simple. It can be done at home, or at work, or wherever you spend a good deal of your time.

What are the requirements for sprouting?

Warmth, moisture and thorough rinsing.

How are the sprouts used in the diet?

They may be eaten alone or with a salad, but should never be cooked.

THE PROPER FOODS TO EAT

SWEET FRUIT

Banana	Date	Papaya
Carob	Fig	Raisin
Cherimoya	Grape, Sweet	Sapote
Cherry	Persimmon	
Currant	Mango	

SUB ACID FRUIT

Apple	Grape, Sour	Pear
Apricot	Blueberry	Plum
Blackberry	Huckleberry	Sapodilla
Elderberry	Nectarine	
Gooseberry	Peach	

ACID FRUIT

Grapefruit	Orange	Quince
Guava	Pineapple	Raspberry
Kumquat	Lime	Strawberry
Loganberry	Tomato	Tamarind
Lemon	Pomegranate	Tangerine

- Avocado (an excellent fruit rich in fat) is best eaten with vegetables.
- Melons (all kinds) should be eaten alone.

MELONS

Banana Melon	Cranshaw melon	Nutmeg melon
Canteloupe	Honeydew melon	Persian melon
Casaba	Muskmelon	Watermelon
Christmas melon		

PROTEINS

Almonds	Peanuts*	Sesame seeds
Cashew nuts	Pecans	Soy bean
Coconut	Pine nuts	Sunflower seeds
Hazel nuts	Pistachio Nuts	Walnuts
Lentils*		

* Peanuts, lentils, beans and all cereals are considered as protein and starch combinations.

STARCHES

Artichoke	Corn	Peas
Bean (lima)*	Hubbard squash	Potatoes
Beets	Jerusalem	Pumpkin
Chestnut	artichoke	Yam
Carrots	Peanuts*	(sweet potato)

NON STARCHY VEGETABLES

Bamboo shoot	Eggplant	Okra
Broccoli	Endive	Parsnips
Brussel sprouts	Kale	Pepper (sweet)
Cabbage	Kohlrabi	Turnip
Cauliflower	Lettuce	(mildly starchy)
(mildly starchy)	—Boston	Rutabaga
Celery	—Romaine	(mildly starchy)
Chard	—Limestone	Squash
Cucumber	—Leaf	(mildly starchy)

For a more complete list of good foods read Dr. William Esser's "Dictionary of Man's Foods."

Combining Foods Properly

There are sound physiological reasons for eating foods in compatible combinations. In other words, some foods, if mixed in the digestive system, will cause distress!

The principles of food combining are dictated by digestive chemistry.

Different foods are digested differently. Starchy foods require an alkaline digestive medium which is supplied initially in the mouth by the enzyme ptyalin. Protein foods require an acid medium for digestion—hydrochloric acid.

As any student of chemistry will assure you, acids and bases (alkalis) neutralize each other. If you eat a starch with a protein, digestion is impaired or completely arrested! The undigested food mass can cause various kinds of digestive disorders. Undigested food becomes soil for bacteria which ferment and decompose it. Its by-products are poisonous, one of which, alcohol, is a narcotic that destroys or inhibits nerve function. It plays havoc with nerves of the digestive tract, suspending their vital action such that constipation may well be a result!

As set forth in Dr. Herbert Shelton's FOOD COMBINING MADE EASY these are the salient rules for proper food combining.

1. Eat acids and starches at separate meals. Acids neutralize the alkaline medium required

for starch digestion and the result is fermentation and indigestion.

2. Eat protein foods and carbohydrate foods at separate meals. Protein foods require an acid medium for digestion.

3. Eat but one kind of protein food at a meal.

4. Eat proteins and acid foods at separate meals. The acids of acid foods inhibit the secretion of the digestive acids required for protein digestion. Undigested protein putrefies in bacterial decomposition and produces some potent poisons.

5. Eat fats and proteins at separate meals. Some foods, especially nuts, are over 50% fat and require hours for digestion.

6. Eat sugars (fruits) and proteins at separate meals.

7. Eat sugars (fruits) and starchy foods at separate meals. Fruits undergo no digestion in the stomach and are held up if eaten with foods that require digestion in the stomach.

8. Eat melons alone. They combine with almost no other food.

9. Desert the desserts. Eaten on top of meals they lie heavy on the stomach, requiring no digestion there, and ferment. Bacteria turn them into alcohols and vinegars.

This is a brief review of the reasons for careful food combining. I urge you to read Dr. Herbert M. Shelton's *Food Combining Made Easy* for a rather thorough treatment of this subject.

FOOD COMBINING FOR EASIEST DIGESTION

One food at a meal is the most ideal for the easiest and best digestion. Combination of several foods at a meal should be according to the chart below. A meal should not consist of more than four foods.

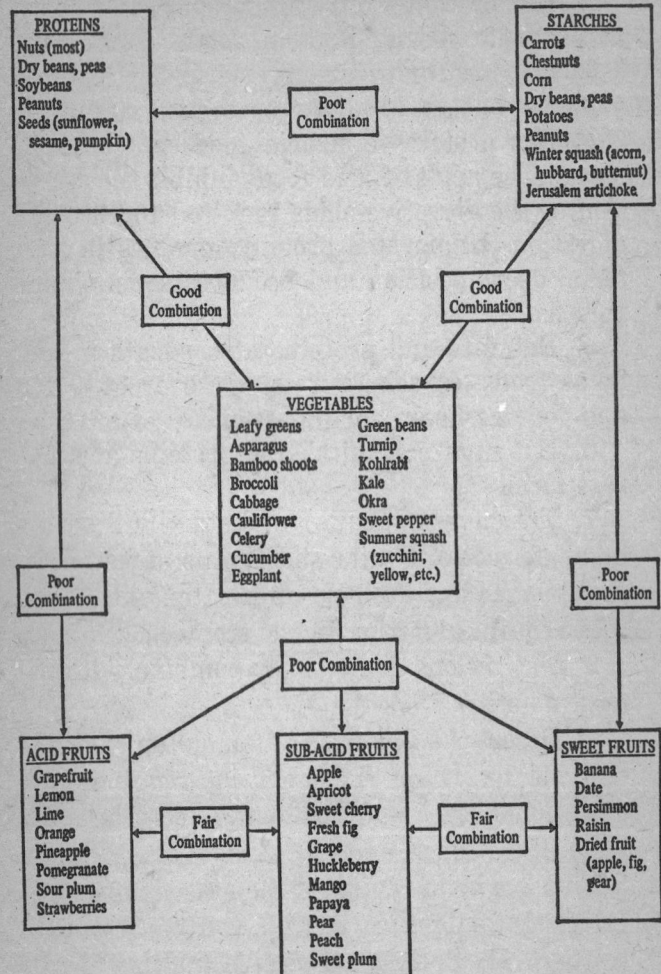

Avocados, rich in fat, are best combined with green vegetables.
Tomatoes may be best eaten with non-starchy vegetables and proteins.
Melons (all kinds) should be eaten alone.

Diet Principles to Follow That Do Not Cause Acid Indigestion, Upset Stomach, Constipation, Heartburn, Digestive Disorders, Etc.

It is not within the scope of this publication to dwell adequately upon the principles enunciated here. If you review them frequently in conjunction with related material in this booklet and other hygienic literature, you'll improve your digestion such that you'll live in perfect harmony and peace with your alimentary system! Instead of it being a battleground often growling back at you and imposing its miseries, you'll hardly ever be aware of its existence! It will function as quietly and inobtrusively as, say, your pituitary glands of which you can hardly be conscious of.

The rules for proper eating are as follows:

1. Eat only when hungry. Don't confuse hunger with appetency.

2. Eat only when free of emotional stress. Eat when calm, relaxed, rested, unworried and unhurried. Never eat when sick, in pain, angry, frustrated or upset. As a hygienist you should not be beset by these latter states.

3. Do not drink immediately before, during or after meals! Drinks interfere with the digestive fluids. A wholesome diet is water-sufficient and, under most circumstances, you'll never drink at all, water or anything else! Your writer has gone up to a month without so much as a sip of any liquid! As you'll learn, most drinking is a pathological and pathogenic practice!

4. Eat only foods that agree with you, that is, delicious foods that cause no problems. Eat only foods that, if eaten alone, are delicious and that can be relished for their own sake until you've had your fill.

5. Eat only fruits, nuts, vegetables and selected seeds.

6. Eat only living foods, that is, foods in their "raw" or natural state. Cooked and processed foods are dead foods. Dead foods make dull, listless lackluster people with much disease and suffering. Perk up your life with living foods.

7. Eat only whole unprocessed, uncooked natural foods while they're fresh, luscious and tasty. Keep in mind that, unspoiled by cooking, processing and other tampering, foods have their nutrients intact and most foods are complete enough in their nutrients to furnish a wide range of human requirements. For example, two or three apples, three or four bananas, a sweet potato or two, furnish the basis for a rather complete meal in themselves though, in the case of the sweet potato, hy-

gienists would supplement it with a green salad.

8. Eat a hearty green salad every day on which you are partaking of a full dietary. Especially good are such greens as kale, cabbage, alfalfa and bean sprouts, celery, broccoli and all lettuces excepting iceberg.

9. As a rule skip breakfast, that is, the morning meal. Breakfast is actually the first meal of the day that "breaks the fast" no matter when eaten. A morning meal is the most unnecessary meal of the day! The body has been assimilating the previous day's food all night and requires nothing further!

10. MASTICATE YOUR FOOD THOROUGHLY! The more you chew your food the more surface area you give its particles thus exposing it more to the digestive juices. The more you chew it the more you ensalivate it and the quicker it will digest and become food for you rather than soil for the bacterial flora in your system which will ferment or putrefy it.

11. DON'T OVEREAT! Eat well within your digestive capacity. Excess food is not digested and is soil for bacterial decomposition. Eat just enough to maintain your ideal weight. Don't worry about little pluses or minuses in your ideal weight level. Therefore, eat as little as you possibly can—not as much as you can. Americans habitually eat 2 or 3 times the quantity of food they require. Reduce your food intake and you'll be healthier!

12. Eat your foods in compatible combinations. See the chapter herein on food combin-

ing principles. Incompatible foods make a battleground out of your stomach instead of a source of sustenance.

13. Eat at room temperature! Hot foods destroy digestive enzymes and cold foods render digestive enzymes inactive. Hot foods destroy living cells by the millions! Why scald your insides?

14. Eat at least 80% of your foods that are alkaline in metabolic reaction. In fact the dietary recommended by NATURAL HYGIENE is over 90% alkaline as actually consumed so there is no worry on this score. Cooked and pasteurized foods will cause harmful acid end products in metabolism whereas the same foods would not in their natural state.

15. DO NOT eat meats, eggs, milks or any animal foods. Do not eat any grain or grain products (such as bread and cereals) except fresh corn and, possibly, as sprouted grains. All these foods are acid-forming and unsuited to the human alimentary system. The human digestive system adapted itself to a frugivorous dietary over an immense span of time, millions of years, and this adaptation must be respected if we are to enjoy optimum health and wellbeing. You cannot expect cattle to change from grass which is a complete food for them to the flesh of animals. Their adaptation is to grasses.

16. NEVER ingest condiments of any kind. This means no salt, spices, pepper, (any kind except sweet pepper which is a food, not a condiment), vinegars, seasonings, onions, gar-

lic, mustard, catsup, etc. These substances interfere with digestion, even stop it! Whole foods taste sufficiently good in themselves to undepraved appetites. Only cooked foods and foods not natural to the human palate require these substances to render them acceptable to our taste buds. Condiments mask unwholesome foods and flavors, give ersatz satiation in place of nutrients robbed from foods, notably mineral salts. ANYTHING you cannot relish with gusto without condiments SHOULD NOT BE EATEN!

17. Allow at least five hours between meals. Two meals a day, one at noon, the other in the evening, is best. Clear your digestive system and give it a rest before giving it new digestive tasks.

18. Eat only in pleasant surroundings and among pleasant people. Upsetting surroundings and upsetting people mean upset stomach!

19. Rest after you've eaten! Don't engage in exercise or rigorous activity. About 25% of your blood supply and energies are required for digestion. Don't impair your digestive processes.

20. While these rules will always improve your digestion if followed, in themselves they cannot assure best digestion. Only in conjunction with a complete health-generating regimen such as is set forth under the 18 essential health factors and influences can good digestion and, consequently, good health be fully realized.

How To Increase The Nutritional Value of Your Food Several Hundred Percent By A Simple Change In The Way You Eat It!

The change is simple indeed: Don't eat cooked or fractured foods!

The eating of cooked food is practically universal and it is, therefore, safe to assume that you eat cooked foods.

COOKED FOODS ARE INHERENTLY PATHOGENIC!

Why?

Cooking destroys 100% of the vital force of foods, that is, their enzymes, auxones, hormones plus food factors only hinted at, as yet, by research. They are, therefore, deficient as foods.

Heat destroys up to 100% of the vitamin content of foods. From the moment heat is applied the reduction from a wholesome food to a poisonous ash has begun. Almost all foods are replete with a whole array of vitamins as well as innumerable enzymes and other food factors. Cooking destroys them from the moment heat is applied and, if applied long enough, DESTROYS THEM ALL!

Cooking de-aminizes proteins and renders them inappropriable by the human economy.

Cooking converts starches to simple sugars and then caramelizes them.

Cooking changes food oils and fats to indigestible and poisonous substances.

Cooking renders minerals from their colloidal organic form to their native inorganic state. Inorganic minerals are not digestible or assimilable by the body economy. Instead of fulfilling vital body needs they become unwelcome poisons in the system. The residue of burning is a blackened ash—thoroughly poisonous—proof enough that any part of the minerals reduced to ash in the cooking process are also poisonous.

IF YOU CAN'T EAT A FOOD IN ITS NATURAL OR "RAW" STATE DON'T! There are enough fine foods that you can eat in their natural state, that is, "alive" or "raw" without resorting to foods you think you need.

Man's biological heritage dictates his dependence upon natural foods that are in no way tampered with by processing, heat, etc. You will do well to follow those practices which are in accord with our natural adaptation.

You can, therefore, increase the value of the food you ingest immeasurably SIMPLY BY EATING IT IN ITS LIVING STATE JUST AS NATURE YIELDS IT UP TO US.

Why You Should Not Eat Bread—Any Kind

The first objection TO ANY BREAD is that it must be cooked! This makes it a dead food as opposed to a living food and dead foods make dead people! Slowly dead, to be sure, but dead nevertheless long before true life potential has been realized and with much suffering along the way.

Besides this evil, breads involve, usually, fracture foods, that is foods so fragmented and separated from their nutrients that they are, in effect, fuel only and little enough of that. They represent abominable combinations, so much so, they are bound to occasion indigestion; fermentation, putrefaction or both. The body seeks simple, not complex digestive tasks!

It is outside the purview of this book to treat exhaustively the gross evils of all cooked foods, fractured and fragmented foods, atrocious combinations of foods, etc. but the pointers furnished herein should be taken heed of!

Bread has been expunged forever from the dietary of the true hygienist.

Why Babies Should Not Be Fed Cereals!

Most American physicians who practice pediatrics ignorantly prescribe cereals, starchy and other solid foods for infants when they are some two or three months old. Never was a greater dietetic error committed! It is a crime against children to be fed starches before . . .

Babies do not secrete the starch-splitting enzyme, ptyalin, until after they have teeth! This enzyme is absent from their saliva until then. Starches should not be fed to babies and to do so before they are biologically ready for them is to seriously impair and injure their health! Without the enzyme ptyalin starches cannot be digested! In a baby's stomach starches become sour, that is, they ferment, form vinegars and alcohols. Starches become the soil for bacterial decomposition in baby's stomach rather than food it can utilize.

The forcing of foods into a baby which is physiologically unsuited to it begins a life of dietetic depravity and perversion, a life of disease, physical debility and suffering.

Babies wisely spit out foods not suited to them. They balk, refuse to eat and then spit out unsuitable foods. Babies aren't contrary—

they're guided by body intelligence born of instinct and body chemistry. Only under great protest will babies finally ingest the bestial "foods" prescribed for them and which are literally forced into them.

It is no wonder that babies cry, are cantankerous, have stomach pains, indigestion, colic, vomiting, fevers, colds, foul stools, etc. Their loving mothers are forcing upon them a diet regimen prescribed by an almost universally ignorant medical profession! Ill health is visited upon babies by those who seek, above all things, health for babies!

Is it any wonder that, wrongly fed and wrongly guided that 58.6% of our children cannot pass a minimum physical fitness test? That cancer is the number one killer of our children? That obesity is so common among children as to cause no alarm? That the average child has such bad teeth it is criminal?

Mothers who love their children can find no better way to care for their children than hygienic care. The Society publishes an excellent book by Dr. Herbert M. Shelton, THE HYGIENIC CARE OF CHILDREN, which should be MUST READING for all mothers and mothers-to-be.

Why Salt Should Never Be Used

There are only *THREE*, count them, THREE inorganic nutrients the body can utilize. These are:

1. Pure Water
2. Pure Air
3. Sunshine

Remember this IN ALL CASES! There is nothing that is inorganic that can be assimilated by the body other than these. Synthetics are an abomination to the body regardless of so-called scientific statements (should be read as "commercial" statements) because the body rejects them!

SALT, sodium chloride, is inorganic! It is NOT a nutrient. It is an irritant and a poison. It is not digested in the body. It becomes saline and is held in solution. The body cannot use it. Under no circumstances does the body use it! No animal in nature needs salt, all the myths to the contrary! It is a poison and an ounce or two taken at once will lay us to rest forever. (We may hold several ounces in our body in solution if we are salt-eaters.)

Everything man takes into his stomach is either a food or a poison! Most poisons are ejected. Some are not ejected fully. Some are retained and "put under the rug", tucked away in the body where they offer the least harm.

Salt is a poison that the body keeps building up until it causes many discomforts and diseases, edema being one of its lesser complaints. It has been indicated as the primary or contributing cause in almost all cases of cancer, heart disease, heart congestion, high blood pressure and other maladies!

Salt is deadly poisonous to children. In a Rochester, New York hospital in the mid-fifties a nurse mistakenly added salt instead of sugar to the milk formula with the result that several infants died and others were seriously ill.

Salt, in solution, is injected into the veins of pregnant women to cause abortion.

Salt will cause vomiting, bowel action, heart acceleration and other body emergency actions. Salt in the system robs body cells of their liquids!

Salt addiction has been with man as far as we can determine ONLY since he started cooking his foods, that is, devitalizing them with heat. Salt restores in part the taste of the natural salts (NOT SODIUM CHLORIDE), which foods are robbed of in cooking but IT DOES NOT RESTORE THE LOST MINERAL NUTRIENTS!

The Indians of America did not use salt—in fact almost no primitive peoples who subsisted upon living ("raw") foods ever used it.

Salt is a poison whether it is sea salt, mined or otherwise manufactured. Under no circumstances should you ever take it into your system!

The body uses *many* salts including sodium chloride but ONLY when in ORGANIC form as found in plant life. These are variously called vegetable or mineral salts.

Shun salt. IT IS HARD NOT TO GET ENOUGH if you partake of the diet advocated by the HYGIENIC SYSTEM.

Salt is not an aid to taste but masks true taste!

Once your taste buds are returned to normalcy you'll never miss salt and will, in fact discover flavors in foods that you never realized existed before!

It is estimated that upwards of 300,000 people annually *drown* because of excess fluids in the body—fluids that are there because of salt! An ounce of salt in the body will require about three quarts of water to hold it in solution. A salt-eater that has about four ounces of salt in his system will carry with him three gallons of water, therefore. This is 24 pounds.

People who appear obese, fat or bloated usually can slim down nicely in a matter of days merely by discontinuing the salt habit! The salt habit can be easily discontinued by eating foods sufficient in mineral salts. THIS MEANS *UNCOOKED FOODS*, FOODS THAT ARE ALIVE AND UNROBBED OF THEIR INHERENT MINERAL SALTS OF WHICH ORGANC SODIUM CHLORIDE IS ONLY ONE!

Physicians ignorantly give us "diuretics" to cause urine flow, hopefully to free the body of these liquids. While it is true that these liquids cause internal congestion, cell starvation and poisoning and have a urine-like consistency, but they are not retained in the body because of urinary failure! They are there to hold salt in solution. This is the body's attempt to prevent salt poisoning!

Salt-eaters are heavy drinkers and are likely to have nephritis (Bright's disease) and the use of diuretics is almost sure to bring this kidney disease on!

If you eat salt you're poisoning yourself! Your body cells contract from the irritation, discharge their precious albumen and other vital elements. SALT is one of the causes of hardened tissues, shriveled blood corpuscles, hardened veins and arteries, arthritis and senility!

SALT, being a poison, is an anti-biotic (against life). No bacterial culture can live in a heavy salt solution. It is a pickling agent and an embalming fluid. Salt was and is frequently used to keep meats from "spoiling". It kills bacteria.

The killing process salt inflicts on humans is slow unless huge amounts (an ounce or two at once) are taken. One of the primary causes of glaucoma of the eyes is salt! Blindness is often caused by salt!

After learning that salt was a poison your writer discontinued it instantly. Simultaneously he went on a "living Food" diet consisting only of vegetables, fruits, nuts and seeds. Within three months his weight was down from around 200 to a mere 144! Relatives and friends warned of grave consequences. But, on the same diet, his weight turned around and he gained to a normal weight of around 155 where it has consistently remained for nearly three years.

TAKE A WISE STEP! PROLONG YOUR LIFE!
NEVER EAT SALT IN ANY FORM AGAIN!

How To Increase Your Brainpower and Mental Alertness!

It must be recognized that these improvements are concomitants of general health improvement. This whole booklet is an outline and a program for health improvement.

As Dr. Tilden has observed "A suffering body cripples its mind also". Any body that is impaired in function has its mind similarly affected for all impairments are, in reality, systemic impairments regardless of locale of the specific impairment.

But there are certain mind-sharpening practices you can indulge! After 24 hours or more of fasting the mental faculties focus intensely! Of course there are periods in fasting from about 36 hours to 60 hours when mental faculties may be dulled because of the morbid material thrown into the blood stream during a fast and which circulates through the brain.

If you wish to perform mental feats don't try to do so after meals! There are a few foods that do not dull the mental faculties significantly though eating low calorie foods in small quantities will not dull them noticeably. Such foods require little digestive power and do not throw a heavy load of nutrients into the blood stream. Grapefruit is an example of such food.

There is no food that will sharpen your mental faculties! All foods must undergo digestion and assimilation before any organ can use them.

Improve your health and you'll improve your mental performance!

A Simple Test You Can Make To Determine Your State of Health!

Your blood stream is the transportation system for your body. Your heart is the workhorse that enables the blood to carry out its physiological tasks of supplying the body's some 25 trillion cells and carrying away their waste matters—even the cells themselves when they are replaced. The brain is the "computer center" that directs the whole body operation from stem to stern.

You can measure the status of your health by determining the workload of your internal transportation system. (This is generally true —there are exceptions.)

The workload of your bloodstream can be determined by counting your pulse.

As a rule the more toxic your system the greater the body's workload. The brain has chemically sensitive instruments which determine the amount of toxic matter in the blood stream and increases or decreases the pumping rate of the heart in ratio of requirements to sustain a physiologically livable blood composition.

To determine if you have a pathological or a healthy pulse keep in mind the faster your heart beats, as a rule, the more toxic is your system. When we run or indulge in vigorous exercise the increased carbon dioxide of the blood accelerates heart function to pass off this waste through the lungs. Faster blood circulation that results from exercise also increases the supply of oxygen and blood sugar to cells that have expended their supplies. After exercise has begun your pulse shoots up and, usually, within a few minutes, it returns to "normal", the toxic load created after its cessations by the exercise having been reduced and the depleted cell supplies having been replenished.

In a state of rest the healthier you are the lower your pulse will be.

The greatest athletes have resting pulses with counts of 30 to 40 beats per minute!

Physicians regard as normal a pulse of 72 beats per minute! This is a pathological rate!

While not "scientifically" established your editor thinks that, ideally, the pulse of a man at rest should be in the 40 to 50 range and that of a woman 6 to 8 beats higher. A child will normally have a pulse about 10 beats higher per minute than its adult counterpart.

Normal daily activities increase the pulse count about 8 to 12 beats per minute. Your editor regards as reflective of a relatively good state of health the following pulse rates:

IN A STATE OF REST

ADULT MALE	40 to 50 pulse beats per minute
ADULT FEMALE	46 to 56 pulse beats per minute
CHILD, MALE	50 to 60 pulse beats per minute
CHILD, FEMALE	56 to 66 pulse beats per minute

IN A NORMAL ACTIVE STATE

ADULT MALE	50 to 60 pulse beats per minute
ADULT FEMALE	56 to 66 pulse beats per minute
CHILD, MALE	60 to 70 pulse beats per minute
CHILD, FEMALE	66 to 76 pulse beats per minute

Higher pulse beats are to be expected after vigorous exercise or after meals when the blood stream is heavily involved in digestion. Also the pulse may increase normally during the early part of our daily cycle when the body is in a predominantly eliminative phase. This is usually from about 3:00 AM to about 7:00 AM or even later.

If we ingest foods which the physiological mechanism recognizes or treats as toxic (this is said to be an allergic food) the pulse will shoot up to as much as 100% above normal!

Cooked foods and unwholesome foods will cause a pathologically high pulse beat and this is primarily responsible for the abnormally high pulse beat regarded as normal by physicians.

A low pulse is not always an indicator of good health but a non-ceasing rapid pulse beat is invariably an indicator of a pathological organism.

The "PULSE TEST" is, therefore, a rather reliable barometer of our state of health.

Questions and Answers on Natural Hygiene

Q. Why is NATURAL HYGIENE a true system of health care?

A. Because it bases its program upon the use of those elements and influences man has become dependent upon for well-being through millions of years of adaptation and development while a creature of nature.

Q. How does NATURAL HYGIENE keep me healthy?

A. By following the NATURAL HYGIENE program *you will* keep yourself healthy in two ways:
   1. By supplying your body with the elements and influences established as being essential to health and ....
   2. By avoiding or not indulging those factors and influences established as being injurious to health, that is, causing illness.

Q. How does NATURAL HYGIENE help me if I am sick?

A. As a follower of NATURAL HYGIENE you should not become sick but, if you do, you'll remove the cause of affliction and, through physiological rest (fasting), enable your body to devote its full restorative powers to healing itself.

Q. What causes most sickness?

A. Failure of the body to expel metabolic wastes and unwelcome substances sufficiently, thus resulting in harmful accumulations. (Read Dr. Tilden's book "TOXEMIA EXPLAINED.")

Q. Aren't diseases caused by germs?

A. No! Germs are no more a cause of disease than flies are a cause of garbage, and for the same reason!

When we speak of germs, microbes or viruses we really mean bacteria, a weak form of parasitic plant life. They serve as nature's scavengers, i.e., they decompose or ferment dead material. They are impotent against living cells.

At most bacteria are a complicating factor in disease but only after the conditions of the disease ALREADY EXIST! Once our waste matters accumulate and our cells die, bacteria decompose them and the by-products of bacterial decomposition are poisonous to our system. According to Koch's postulate, if germs are a cause of disease they must always be present if the disease they cause exists (Much of the time they are not!) and if the germs are present they must always cause the disease of their peculiarity. (And they are frequently present in individuals without causing the disease for which they are ascribed as agency!)

Man is dependent upon bacteria for many of his functional needs, for example, the making of Vitamin B-12. As long as we maintain ourselves through good health practice we have absolutely nothing to fear from "germs".

Q. Why do waste materials and poisons accumulate in the body?

A. Either because we overload the body beyond its eliminative capacity or because a lowered fund of nerve energy is incapable of maintaining the normal processes of excretion.

Q. What causes loss of sufficient nerve energy?

A. An unnatural pattern of living that expends this vital force beyond our bodies ability to regenerate it through rest and sleep. When we have expended this miracle of life we are said to be in a state of nervous exhaustion.

Q. What are some examples of unnatural living?

A. Insufficient rest and sleep, too little or too much physical activity, stress, overeating or eating unnatural foods, lack of sunshine and light, use of coffee, tobacco, alcohol, drugs, stimulants, etc.

How Over 200 Million Americans Are Hooked on Drugs and Don't Realize It!

Americans cry to high heaven about their drug problem! But they actually are decrying the practices of just a few Americans, a few hundred thousand who take heroin, LSD, Opium, Cocaine, Marijuana and other such esoteric drugs labelled "hard drugs"!

They overlook that America, at large, has a *drug culture!* THEY OVERLOOK ALMOST ENTIRELY THE REAL DRUG PROBLEM THAT INVOLVES ALMOST EVERY LAST AMERICAN!

The drugs doing the most harm in America are:

1. Nicotine (this is but one of 16 poisons in tobacco!)

2. Caffeine (from coffee, colas and other drinks, foods and drugs!)

3. Alcohol (in liquors, wines, beers, miscellaneous drinks!)

4. Vinegar (a commonly used condiment that is a first cousin to alcohol!)

5. Alcohol (as a by-product of fermentation in our digestive systems!)

6. Aspirin (salicylic acid)
7. Salt (all salt!)
8. Theine (in teas and certain herbal drinks—akin to caffeine)
9. Theobromine (in cocoa and chocolate products—akin to caffeine)
10. Sugar (though not regarded as a drug, generally, it produces the effects of drugs!)
11. Every drug in the pharmacopoeia! There are thousands of them and physicians issue over a billion drug prescriptions a year! *Millions* of Americans are addicted to barbiturates, amphetamines, tranquilizers, (these addictions begin primarily upon the prescriptions of physicians), and what have you!

NICOTINE is perhaps the most lethal of the poisons Americans indulge as a matter of practice. It is a NARCOTIC just as much as such so-called hard drugs as heroin, morphine, opium, etc. Because it has a long-standing history and a huge industry thrives upon this deadly drug it has achieved respectability! In other words tobacco is a legalized narcotic!

Tobacco has 16 specific poisons and inhaling ANY KIND OF SMOKE adds a train of other harmful poisons—tars and oxidation products! All coat and clog the lungs, thus reducing our capacity for oxygen assimilation and, worse, causing us to retain greater amounts of respiratory excreta in our systems!

Every tobacco smoker is, whether he realizes it or not, a *drug addict*, A NARCOTIC AD-

DICT if you please, committing a slow painful suicide!

CAFFEINE is a habit forming stimulant that causes the body to act just the opposite of nicotine. While nicotine depresses, subdues or lowers vital action through nerve paralysis or narcotization, caffeine accelerates or increases vital action. It does not increase nerve activity by furnishing nutrients required by the nervous system or any other bodily structure. On the contrary caffeine occasions stepped up activity in the body—an eliminative activity. Caffeine is equally obnoxious and almost as poisonous as nicotine. In the human system caffeine causes accelerated activity to the end that the offending substance, caffeine, be expelled.

That which causes stepped up body activity is called a stimulant. The body is stimulated because it accelerates its vital functions (at a great expense to its fund of nerve energy) to reject *all* non-utilizable and harmful substances introduced into it if that substance does not, first, as in the case of nicotine and other narcotics, form chemical unions that lower, inhibit or destroy nerve function.

HOW MANY AMERICANS REGULARLY USE THE DRUG CAFFEINE? Almost all of us including our children right down to the ages of two or three!

CAFFEINE is a common substance in coffee, all soft drinks advertised as colas and it is added to others—in fact soft drinks usually introduce more caffeine into our systems than do an equivalent amount of coffee! Caffeine is put into many products today to "give them zip", EVEN ICE CREAM! To avoid this pathogenic product don't eat ANY processed food! Avoid all soft drinks! In fact a water sufficient diet of fruits, vegetables, nuts and seeds in their *natural* state is insurance against this and other poisonous products that are added to our foods as a matter of course.

ALCOHOL is another narcotic! It is also a *legalized* narcotic! Every alcoholic is, therefore, a narcotic addict! Alcohol is the toxic by-product of bacterial fermentation and is poisonous to both bacteria and man alike! It is poisonous to our animal brethren too! Alcohol is the noxious excreta of bacterial activity on certain types of substances, notably the starch family of foods. It is an anti-biotic. It is a preservative. It is an antiseptic. And it is always poisonous to the human system to varying degrees in relation to its kind and quantity! Methyl alcohol is lethal in even small quantities.

In the human body it destroys nerve and brain cells! Alcohol is addictive, that is, habit forming as is coffee, tobacco and the cola drinks. The principal sources of alcohol for Americans are in whiskies and liquors, beers and wines— where alcohol is procured as such. But there is a greater source of alcohol . . . . . . !

Perhaps half of us are unintentional alcoholics!

Unfortunately the most dedicated opponent

of alcohol in social life can be an alcoholic—an unintentional alcoholic!

Alcohols are made from sugar, potatoes, fruits, grains such as wheat, corn, barley, rice and other starches and carbohydrates. Alcohol is the by-product of fermentation of these food substances.

When we eat these foods in their natural state, that is, with their enzymes and other reproductive factors intact as found in their "raw" state, their breakdown is rapid in our systems because the inherent enzymes break the food down rapidly at body temperatures and it is thus the more rapidly digested and assimilated. But, even then, if the food is combined with incompatible foods or substances such that digestion is held up, fermentation is likely! But . . . .

But if these foods are cooked and rendered dead foods and then eaten, especially in conjunction with other foods or substances that retard digestion, bacteria have a Roman holiday! Result: Alcohol! Alcohol is absorbed by our system in mild form and we are thus mildly narcotized.

Perhaps most of us are familiar with birds that eat grains and grass seeds and then eat fruits, especially cherries, on top of it. They really and truly become drunk! They're drunk on the alcohol they formed in their own intestinal systems.

There are untold millions of such inebriates in America today! That is why . . . .

SUGAR should be classified as a drug! The average American takes in about four ounces daily. It is taken in as a sweetener—it is in about everything. In the unphysiological combinations in which it is ingested and because of the great difficulty of breaking down sucrose in most systems anyway, it is held up until it ferments and the by-product of sugar fermentation is alcohol. A sugar addict may well be an alcohol addict!

Sugar, of course, is a totally dead substance. It has been cooked, retorted, extracted and refined to death. It is without even a semblance of usable nutrients. It has only caloric value. Taken into the body it robs the body of nutrients the body already possesses! It requires alkaline elements, especially calcium as in our teeth and bones, to neutralize its acid end products.

Remember—sugar is deadly and the person who "craves" sugar as millions do is, undoubtedly, an alcoholic without knowing it.

VINEGAR is a first cousin to alcohol! Both are the poisonous and indigestible excreta of bacteria. Both make excellent preservatives and both are anti-biotics. Because vinegar is acidic and has a flavor derived from the plant which was decomposed (fermented) to obtain it, there are many different flavors of vinegar, e.g., apple cider, sauerkraut, grape, berry, etc. Wine, an alcoholic, is obtained by only a slightly different fermentation process than vinegar.

Vinegar has won favor as a condiment but

has no virtues on that account. It is unwelcome in the human body.

Not only is vinegar indigestible but it renders other foods indigestible for it neutralizes the base digestive juices, destroys intestinal flora because of its anti-biotic qualities and, because of its noxious properties, occasions a more rapid expulsion of the stomach's contents.

Vinegar deserves to be classed as a drug for it contains no nutrient qualities whatsoever derivable by the body and it is harmful in the human system. Fortunately, we take very little vinegar at any one time.

ASPIRIN is a drug that may be obtained without prescription and is taken for numerous complaints, primarily headache. It is a nervine, a nice way of saying it paralyzes the nerves through chemical unions. It is a favorite for headaches.

Taking away the ability of the nerves to register body distress no more removes body distress than removing a thermometer changes room temperature! Thus aspirin could well be called an oral anesthetic! It does not remove the headache—it renders us incapable of longer feeling the headache. That blessed relief is the same kind of relief a narcotic addict gets from indulging his opium or heroin!

SALT is one of the most pernicious of drugs. It is poisonous and indigestible in the human system. It is used by physicians to cause abortions through its injection as a saline solution into the veins of pregnant women. It is an excellent anti-biotic for it is deadly to bacteria. You'll find this insidious condiment treated at length elsewhere.

THEINE is a poisonous stimulant found in most teas that we drink in America, especially the favorite teas which we give to even the smallest tots with lemon and sugar! THEINE is nothing more than our old friend, caffeine, all over again! Only in tea it is called theine. The manifold evils born of caffeine ingestion apply equally to theine.

THEOBROMINE is a poison taken by most AMERICANS! Here is the definition of theobromine taken from the Random House dictionary: "A poisonous powder, used chiefly as a diuretic, myocardial stimulant and vasodilator. Found in genus of trees typified by cacao."

Theobromine is a deadly drug and it is the bitter substance in cocoa! Americans innocently get this stimulating poison (stimulating because it occasions stepped up body activity to get it out the system as fast as possible) in chocolate products, cocoa drinks, ice creams, candies, etc. EVEN BABIES ARE GIVEN THIS DANGEROUS DRUG! Combined with sugar to disguise its bitterness (its obnoxious poison is not palatable except in disguise) chocolate is regarded as America's number one confection! It could be called America's NUMBER ONE DRUG! The eating of chocolate products is nearly universal. Actually, though not regarded as drugs, salt and sugar stand at the front of America's drug habits!

Chocolate stands third on the list of allergenic substances! The body is quite properly allergic to poisons! Milk is first on the list of allergies and wheat is second. You'll do well to study why not only milk and wheat are, in effect, drugs in many humans but why many other common "foods" are nothing but deleterious substances in the human organism.

Each year about 4,500,000 persons in the U.S.A. are poisoned so seriously *BY THEIR OWN PHYSICIANS* that they require hospitalization! Such persons have been said to have had "adverse reactions" or undesired "side effects" from their medicines. This is perfumed language for "poison effects"! ALL DRUGS ARE INHERENTLY POISONOUS!

KEEP THIS IN MIND! ONLY WHOLESOME NUTRITIOUS FOODS SHOULD PASS BEYOND OUR LIPS! ANYTHING TAKEN INTO THE BODY OTHERWISE IS A SYSTEMATIC POISON AND NO POISON CAN BENEFIT US! Even food taken in unwholesome combinations or inordinate amounts can cause poisoning!

DRUGS ARE DEADLY! SHUN THEM ALL FROM WHATEVER SOURCE! I trust that you can now see how almost EVERY AMERICAN is hooked on one or more drug habits.

Do Drugs or "Medicines" Really Cure?

Space permits only a very simple response to this question. The answer is No! There are NO CURES WHATSOEVER FROM ANY SOURCE!

An ailing or diseased body requires healing—physiological correction! All healing is a biological process AND ONLY THE AFFECTED ORGANISM HAS IN IT THE POWER TO HEAL! There are no other healing powers. The capacity to heal is inherent in the organism.

Diseases are symptoms of bodily healing crises. They are an evidence of vital action to expel morbid matters and to restore normal function.

Drugs furnish no nutrients. They have no intelligence to create new cells and repair damaged tissue. Instead drugs form chemical unions that paralyze nerves and suspend vital action, thus suppressing symptoms of disease. The person thus treated is sicker than before even though appearing and feeling better!

Drugs which have a stimulant action rather than a narcotic action goad the body into extraordinary eliminative activity but this exhausts an already exhausted body thus resulting in the subject being worse off than before.

All healing that takes place after the administration of drugs (or any other kind of treatment) does so in spite of the drugs, not because of them. Drugs and treatments all rise to glory on the back of the self-healing powers of the body!

Under no circumstances can drugs cure anything and there never will be such a drug. All drugs are inherently poisonous and dangerous to the organism. NO DRUG OF ANY KIND should ever be introduced into the human organism.

Perhaps this subject has never received more illuminating treatment than that given to it by Dr. Herbert M. Shelton. From a past issue of Dr. Shelton's HYGIENIC REVIEW I reproduce one of his articles entitled CURES! CURES! CURES!

Cures! Cures! Cures!

The search for "cures" is older far than the written records of man. Who the first witch-doctor was, history does not record. We do not know when or where he lived. But we do know that he started the race on a search that has never ceased.

No believable estimate can be made of the number of "cures" that have been discovered. When recorded history began, thousands of "cures" were already in use. The medicine men of that time had cures for practically every disease that man suffers with.

But "cures" are peculiar in that they do not long remain cures. New "cures" have to be found to supplant the old ones as these lose their effectiveness. Hence always there has been an army of men and women engaged in the pursuit of new "cures". Perhaps more "cures" have been discovered in man's short historic period than were found through the whole of his long period of pre-history.

Who remembers today the "cures" that were popular ten years ago? Who recalls, except vaguely, the "cures" with which he was treated as a boy in pre-war days? Who can recollect even the names of the popular patent-medicines of twenty and thirty years ago? The "cures" of yester-year are gone. Their places have been filled by many strange "cures" that were unheard of then.

A book on the practice of medicine that is more than two years old is hoary with antiquity. Its "cures" are no longer used. Its pages are filled with forgotten theories and with long discarded "cures". The sober fact is that so rapid is the discovery of new "cures" that the book writers and book publishers cannot get out the books fast enough to keep up with the "advances" of "medical science."

Today the face of the earth is thickly dotted with "research" institutions that are engaged in searching for new "cures". Some of these, like the Rockefeller Institute, are large, heavily endowed institutions filled with every conceivable scientific gadget and staffed by a small army of technically trained men and women. Some are endowed by the various governments. Many are necessary appendages of manufacturing drug houses. Others are small and belong to the ambitious man who vainly searches for some Elixir vitae or some Philosopher's stone.

Perhaps several hundred thousand men and women are engaged in this "research." No believable estimate can be made of the money invested in plant and equipment with which to carry on the mad search for "cures." No one can guess how much money flows into the coffers of the "researchers" to assist in the search for "cures."

Day and night, all over the world, the search

goes on and daily new "cures" are found and heralded to an expectant world; a world that has been taught to look with awe upon the "researcher" and his great stock of knowledge and wisdom. To the discovery of new "cures" there seems to be no end.

The public demands "cures." When the old ones fail, they demand new ones. The cure-mongers demand new "cures." The "researchers" find new "cures." There is always a ready market for "cures" and there seems to be no limit to the amount of money that may be had for "research." The job of the "researcher" is to find "cures" and he finds them. When these fail, he finds new ones.

The drug stores of the world are groaning under their load of "cures"—that do not cure. The mail man brings new "cures" to the physician with almost every mail. The manufacturing drug houses do not permit physicians to remain long in ignorance of the new "cures." Perhaps they remember the words of the famous French physician of the past century, who said to his patient: "Here, take this while it is still a remedy."

Out of all the uncounted millions of "cures" that have been discovered since the first voodoo doctor started mankind on its frenzied hunt for cures, where is there one real cure? Where is the cure for constipation? For indigestion? For colds? For boils? For gastritis? For hives? For pimples? I do not ask for a cure for cancer, for diabetes, or Bright's disease. I ask only for one cure for the simple everyday functional disorders like constipation and indigestion.

In all that vast system of conscious fraud and humbug that proudly styles itself Modern Medical Science, is there one cure for anything? Is there an honest and intelligent physician in the whole world who will claim that he has knowledge of a single cure for even the simplest ailment from which man suffers? If not, is he any less a charlatan than the vilest empiric of the past?

All down the ages there has been a constant and ceaseless change of methods of "curing" coincident with an undying faith in the doctor and his bag of tricks. A credulous public "always comes back for more" cures. If it loses its faith in one vaunted "cure" or to another much advertised school of medicine, it merely transfers its faith to another loudly touted "cure" or to another much advertised school of healing. Its stock of credulity seems never to run out.

If the public is credulous, what must we say about the physicians who are "taken in" by every new "cure" that is offered them by the manufacturing chemists and pharmaceutical supply houses? Do they learn nothing from past failures? If they possessed any real knowledge, would they prescribe and use all the new "cures" offered them by the manufacturers and their subsidized "researchers"? Intelligent and informed men do not "fall" for the same old "gag" repeatedly.

The desire to be "cured" is so strongly imbedded in the average person that he will have a "cure" even if he has to die to get it. Indeed he is usually "cured" repeatedly for the "cures" do not "stay put."

Mr. Average Man believes in treatment. He has been taught from infancy to resort to treatment when ill. The medical professions exist to "treat disease and disorder."

They all believe they can cure disease without removing cause. They are based on a premise as false as the belief that a salve will cure your foot without removing the tack; as false as the belief that a drunk man may be sobered up while he continues to drink.

The discovery, production, distribution and administration of "cures" is a profitable industry. The "research" boys hold down fat, easy jobs. The drug trade pays both the manufacturers and the distributors very well. The physician who administers the various voodoo concoctions is also well paid. The only one who loses by it is the poor sucker who buys the "cure."

A few years ago one of our leading popular weekly magazines estimated that the medical profession had, at that time, over a hundred and thirty thousand "remedies" for the four hundred and seven "diseases" then listed in the medical nosologies. Since that time the number of diseases has been greatly multiplied and the number of "remedies" has been greatly increased. Millions of dollars are invested in the manufacture and distribution of "remedies" and still the human race is sick. With so many "remedies" why should anybody ever remain sick or die "of disease"? If medicine and "curing" is any more than a gigantic and well-paying racket, why don't they cure our "diseases" with their great wealth of "cures"?

Only one thing can cure mankind's belief in "cures". This is knowledge. It is necessary that both physician and layman learn that there are no cures. They must lose their belief in disease; their belief that there are diseases. The belief in disease and cure is the most effective barrier standing between mankind and health.

Knowledge is the greatest need of our benighted and purblind world. Knowledge of how to live; knowledge of the nature and purpose of disease; knowledge of the evils and futility of treatment; knowledge of the truth about life—this is the need of the whole world today.

"My children are killed for lack of knowledge" says the god of the Hebrew scriptures. Millions die yearly because they lack true conceptions of life, of health, of disease, of cure. More people are killed every year by the causes of and the treatments for "disease" than by any other causes, only because their ignorance leads them to ignore causes and to rely upon "cures."

Education must supplant treatment; faith in the processes and forces of life must take the place of faith in "cures"; confidence in the normal things of life must displace confidence in abnormal things; trust in the laws of life must crowd out trust in vicarious atonements. Only thus can the ages-long frenzied search for "cures" be ended. Only thus can the terrible waste of time, money, energy and mental effort in the search for "cures" cease and all this time, money, energy and effort be re-directed into profitable channels.

The frenzied search for "cures" must cease. Mankind must learn that the so-called disease, which they seek to cure, is, itself, the process of cure. All efforts to cure the cure are vicious and destructive. Unfortunately, the "healing" professions and the public still have the troglodyte's conception of disease. They still conceive of it as an attack upon the body by outside and unseen forces. The truth reaches them slowly.

Healing—restoration of health, wholeness, integrity—is a normal, a physiological or biological process. It results from the orderly operations of the ordinary and regular forces and processes of life, working with agents and substances that bear a normal relation to the living organism. Success of the body's efforts at self-healing depends absolutely upon removal of the cause of its ills. This is to say, the body cures itself when cause is removed. There is no cure outside of correction of cause.

Is Natural Hygiene Scientific?

We hygienists contend that NATURAL HYGIENE is, indeed, scientific.

To be scientific means to be true, to be in accord with the facts that appertain.

In matters of health the Society contends that the facts relating to its optimum realization are easy of ascertainment. It contends that the simple health system referred to as NATURAL HYGIENE is in harmony with nature, in accord with the principles of vital organic existence, in agreement with common sense, sound in concept, correct in practice and successful in results.

No other concept that intrudes itself upon the health scene can successfully challenge these contentions.

How, By Following the Hygienic Program, the Average Family Can Save Over $2,000 a Year!

The average American family should realize at least $2,000 extra each year, even if earnings are not increased, by following the hygienic program. These savings can be realized as follows:

1. From the average annual food bill of about $2,600 the average family can save at least $1,000! Yet, to a great extent, the family can eat organically grown foods!

2. America's disease bill in 1973 was about $93,000,000,000 or about $1,800 per family. The average family should be able to save more than $1,000 per year on hospital, doctor, drug and medical related bills! By diligent application of the system of living presented in this publication you can achieve such wonderful health that you'll eliminate nearly the entire amount spent on medical bills. HEALTHY PEOPLE SIMPLY DO NOT NEED PHYSICIANS, DRUGS, HOSPITALS, ETC.! (and neither do sick people!)

3. The hygienic way of living should free the lady of the house of about 500 hours of work

annually! This time saving alone can be worth another $1,000!

4. There are other costs related to the current mode of living, perhaps as much as a thousand dollars, that will be saved on the hygienic regimen.

5. Saving perhaps $3,000 to $4,000 a year is a mere PITTANCE if measured against the greatest benefit of all, SUPERB HEALTH!

NOTICE TO THE READER

If after reading this book, you feel the vital knowledge which it contains deserves to be made widely known, you are urged to become a member of the American Natural Hygiene Society and help to contribute to this worthy cause for the benefit of mankind. (Contributions are tax exempt.)

As a membership bonus, we will send a free copy of this book to anyone of your choice. Fill out the application below and mail with your remittance of $7.00, which includes the annual membership and the bonus book.

AMERICAN NATURAL HYGIENE SOCIETY
1920 IRVING PARK ROAD, CHICAGO, ILL. 60613

Please enroll me as a member of your worthy cause. Enclosed is $7.00 for the Annual Membership and the bonus book.*

Name_____
(please print)

Address_____

City, State, Zip_____

Phone No._____ Age_____

**** PLEASE SEND BONUS BOOK TO ****

Name_____
(please print)

Address_____

City, State, Zip_____

Phone No._____ Age_____

*Outside U.S.A. add $1.00 to cover added postage costs and handling.

BOOK ORDER FORM

- [ ] FASTING FOR RENEWAL OF LIFE — $2.25
- [ ] TOXEMIA: The Basic Cause of All Disease — $1.50
- [ ] PROGRAM FOR DYNAMIC HEALTH — $1.00
- [ ] FASTING CAN SAVE YOUR LIFE — $1.45
- [ ] YOU DON'T HAVE TO BE SICK! — $1.45
- [ ] HEALTH FOR THE MILLIONS — $1.45
- [ ] HYGIENIC CARE OF CHILDREN — $1.95
- [ ] EXERCISE! — $1.95
- [ ] THE GREATEST HEALTH DISCOVERY — $1.75
- [ ] DICTIONARY OF MAN'S FOODS — $2.25
- [ ] SUPERIOR NUTRITION — $2.25
- [ ] INTRODUCTION TO NATURAL HYGIENE — $1.75
- [ ] FOOD COMBINING MADE EASY — $1.00
- [ ] RUBIES IN THE SAND — $4.50
- [ ] SYPHILIS: The Werewolf of Medicine — $4.00
- [ ] LIVING LIFE TO LIVE IT LONGER — $2.00
- [ ] HYGIENIC SYSTEM, Vol. 2 — $5.50
- [ ] HYGIENIC SYSTEM, Vol. 3 — $5.50
- [ ] NATURAL HYGIENE: Man's Pristine Way of Life — $6.50
- [ ] FASTING FOR HEALTH AND LONG LIFE — $3.00
- [ ] HUMAN BEAUTY: ITS CULTURE AND HYGIENE — $10.00

Add 20¢ to each book for postage

Illinois residents add 5% state sales tax.

- [ ] DR. SHELTON'S HYGIENIC REVIEW — $7.50
  (yearly subscription) **Foreign $8.00**
- [ ] FIT FOOD FOR MAN — $.50

American Natural Hygiene Society
1920 Irving Park Road, Chicago, Ill. 60613

Please ship books checked above. Enclosed is $_____

Name_____

Address_____

City, State, Zip_____

WHY NOT RECEIVE A MONTHLY MAGAZINE THAT TELLS THE TRUTH ABOUT HEALTH?

(Subscribe to a magazine that speaks with sanity and intelligence about health)

Dr. Herbert M. Shelton publishes a monthly magazine distributed as the HYGIENIC REVIEW.

Fearless in its defiance of entrenched interests that perpetuate disease to its redounding profit, Dr. Shelton's HYGIENIC REVIEW has been published continuously since September, 1939.

Month after month the HYGIENIC REVIEW brings articles providing unerring guidance in the science of correct living. That truth and sanity might prevail it strikes out boldly and courageously at errors that make their appearance to masquerade on the health scene.

A subscription to this magazine is a MUST!

No other magazine in existence gives such profound unreproachable guidance.

SUBSCRIPTION INFORMATION

A subscription to the HYGIENIC REVIEW costs $7.50 annually for 12 issues. You can send your subscription directly to the Society or to:

HYGIENIC REVIEW
San Antonio, Texas 78295

JOIN OTHERS IN BRINGING HEALTH TO AMERICA

There is much you can do to help bring health to Americans. You can become a member of the American Natural Hygiene Society and thus become a part of a movement that has as its goal the total abolition of disease from America—in fact, the whole human race!

Your membership fee of $7.00 obligates you to nothing. You enjoy several membership benefits, the greatest of which is knowing that you have made it possible for the Society to reach many other people with its message of healthful living.

Other benefits include a subscription to the NATURAL HYGIENE EDUCATOR and to the NATURAL HYGIENE NEWS. These periodicals will keep you abreast of developments within the Society and of its progress in bringing to America the hygienic way of life.

If you elect to become a member and, of course, we urge you to become one, just check off the proper entry on the enclosed SUBSCRIPTION MEMBERSHIP ORDER FORM and remit the sum of $7.00. For further information on additional memberships write to: American Natural Hygiene Society, 1920 Irving Park Road, Chicago, Ill. 60613.

DIRECTORY OF HYGIENIC INSTITUTIONS AND PRACTITIONERS

DR. J. M. BROSIOUS, N.D., D.C.
Bay'n Gulf Hygienic Home
18207-09 Gulf Boulevard
St. Petersburg, Florida 33708
Phone: (813) 392-8326

DR. HERBERT M. SHELTON
Shelton's Health School
RT 10, Box 174E
San Antonio, Texas 78216

DR. VIRGINIA VETRANO
Shelton's Health School
RT 10, Box 174E
San Antonio, Texas 78295
Phone: (512) 697-3613; (512) 438-9293

DR. D. J. SCOTT
Scott's Natural Health Institute
Box 8919
Cleveland, Ohio 44136
Phone: (216) 238-6930

DR. WILLIAM ESSER
Esser's Hygienic Rest Ranch
Box 161
Lake Worth, Florida 33460
Phone: (305) 965-4360

DR. GERALD BENESH
1450 Mission Road
San Marcos, California 92069
Phone: (714) 744-0118